Laurie Pippen's All Natural
Anti-Aging Skin Care Recipe Book

Copyright 2013

Laurie Pippen

The recipes in this book contain easily obtained ingredients that are generally accepted to be safe and effective.

Individual reactions to the contained ingredients can vary. It is not possible to predict how any individual will react to a particular recipe, treatment, or ingredient.

As with any personal care product, common sense should be used when creating these recipes. The reader should consult a qualified physician before using any ingredient or recipe in this book.

The enclosed materials are for informational purposes only and the reader accepts all responsibility for determining the effectiveness and usefulness of all of the included items. Neither the author nor the publisher accepts liability neither for the actions of the reader nor for any reactions caused by the use of the contents and ingredients.

Nothing in this recipe guide is intended to substitute for the medical expertise and advice of your primary health care provider.

You should discuss any decisions about treatment or care with your health care provider. The information contained within this guide is believed to be accurate at the time of writing but research is being undertaken daily and new information, effects, or side effects may be discovered that conflict with the materials contained herein.

No product, service, or therapy is endorsed by the author, publisher, or other individual associated with the creation of this material. The reader should remember that the U.S. Food and Drug Administration (FDA) have not evaluated the statements made in this book. The products listed are not intended to diagnose, treat, cure, or prevent any disease.

Using any medication whether prescription, over the counter, or herbal in nature may have a marked effect on your health and each medicine may interact with others. Tell your health care provider about any complementary, supplemental, or alternative practices you use including dietary substances, herbals, or oils.

Federal regulations for dietary supplements are different from the regulations applied to prescription and over the counter drugs. Dietary supplement manufacturers are not required to prove a product's safety and effectiveness.

Herbs and oils are sometimes marketed as dietary supplements. Herbs and oils do have a noticeable affect on the human body. The expected action of many herbs and oils is based on traditional use and observation. Laboratory studies have been conducted to confirm the expected affect of some traditionally used herbs and oils but others have not been well researched. Most dietary supplements, herbs, and oils have not been researched for use by pregnant women, nursing women, or children. No supplement, herb, or oil in this book is recommended for use by women who are pregnant, nursing, or by children.

Each person's needs and correct dosage will vary depending on a variety of factors. You should discuss your specific needs and best dosage with our physician or qualified herbalist.

Laurie Pippen's
All Natural
Anti-Aging Skin Care Recipe Book

Chapter 1 Aging Skincare.....................................1

Chapter 2 Soaps 3

Chapter 3 Soft Soaps & Cleansers 35

Chapter 4 Exfoliating Scrubs............................55

Chapter 5 Astringents & Toners 71

Chapter 6 Deep Bath Treatments & Masks.......82

Chapter 7 Serums..111

Chapter 8 Lotions and Creams 124

Chapter 9 Mineral Makeup 145

Chapter 10 Natural Ingredients.......................155

Glossary 195

Aging Skin

Normal, healthy skin is a beautiful sight, but aging means that many of us need a little help to keep our skin looking & feeling great.

Skin aging is a natural process that begins almost as soon as we reach adulthood. Each year, our body produces less oil, collagen, and elastin and the skin becomes thinner and more fragile. This internal aging takes place over decades. In most cases, we do not notice dramatic differences in our skin from day to day due to intrinsic aging.

Our skin also ages due to external factors. Exposure to environmental hazards like the sun, pollution, and chemicals can speed skin aging. External aging tends to occur far more quickly and is an area where our actions and care can have a dramatic impact.

There are many simple actions and preventatives you can implement to help improve the look & feel of your skin. You can minimize sun exposure, detoxify your diet, get enough exercise, reduce environmental pollutants like smoking, and hydrate, hydrate, hydrate! A healthy lifestyle can have a dramatic and nearly instant effect on the health of your skin.

In addition to lifestyle changes, you can implement a skin care regimen that addresses the most common types of aging symptoms. Correct skin care can combat the hyper-pigmentation, collagen loss, roughness, thickening, fine lines, deep crevices and other common aging symptoms that occur on our skin because of external factors. The recipes in this book are designed to treat a variety of issues associated with aging including darkening, roughness, uneven tone, and wrinkles ranging from fine lines to deep crevices.

Prevention is the most essential element to minimizing the aging of skin. It is essential that we take action to minimize the affect of environmental aging. Starting a good skin care regimen, whether it is early or late in your life, is critical to how you look & feel every single day.

The recipes in this book help to treat the symptoms of external aging. Each recipe attempts to provide the most effective ingredients. Remember, each person will have a slightly different situation including environment, skin type, personal needs, and history. You should experiment to find the perfect solution for you!

Natural care is about more than just using nature to solve a problem. Natural care is about CUSTOMIZING nature to solve your personal problem!

Soaps

The first step to beautiful, healthy skin is cleansing. You need to find the cleansing products that work best for your particular skin care needs. Before you can use any other product in your regimen the area you are treating must be clean. People sometimes overlook the importance of using the correct soap.

Consider that soap is the first item, and often the last, that you use each day. People often spend the rest of the day using products to counteract the effects of the soap that they have chosen. Using the correct soap can either harm or enhance the results of the rest of your products.

Some people prefer soft soap and that is my favorite method for cleaning my face. Other people prefer a harder soap especially for body care.

Before deciding which soap recipe to try, you should understand the basics of skin and skin care. Many factors can affect the condition and appearance of skin. No soap or other product can replace simple daily care in your activities. Skin is the largest organ you have and perhaps the most important in that it protects every other part of you from environmental factors. Of course, skin is also very important because it is the first thing most people will notice about you.

The type of soap base and customization ingredients used in soap recipes is very specific to the individual. Every person will have slightly different skin care needs. The best way to achieve perfection in your soap-making endeavor is to keep experimenting to determine which soap works best with your skin, lifestyle, and climate.

This chapter outlines the creation of the most common types of soap that you can customize to suit your needs. I have also included a few of my favorite soap customizations for you to use as a starting point. Remember to experiment – most of the ingredients in soap making are extremely cost effective and easy to locate. The more you experiment the more effective the product will be for your specific needs.

Soap recipes are often the most difficult for people to follow. Soap requires more time and effort than most of the other products included in this book. Do not be discouraged by the processes described since soap is a common item that has been successfully created by individuals for generations. To create exceptional soaps you just need to practice and perfect your skills. You will also need some dedicated equipment to create soap. You can easily find these items in specialty craft stores or often in an all-in-one retail chain. Some stores even carry kits that contain most of the key equipment in one package.

Cleansing is one of the best places that you can spend time experimenting and customizing the recipes to suit your needs. The better customized your cleansing regimen is to your particular skin type, lifestyle, and needs the better your appearance will be.

You may need to use different cleansers on different parts of your skin. Face and neck skin tends to be slightly different from the skin on the rest of your body and will need different treatments and preventatives. You should consider the underlying cause of your aging, sensitivity of the areas being treated, and personal application preferences before selecting recipes to try.

Regardless of the recipes you choose to try it is always recommended that you test sample the products on a sensitive area such as your wrist to ensure that you do not have unexpected reactions before applying them to your skin. This is not a fail proof method of ensuring that the products are correct for you but it can often provide a warning of a negative reaction.

Basic Supplies

Thermometer – Successful soap making depends heavily on temperature.

The base components like lye, borax, and fat must be heated to a particular temperature and then cooled to become soap.

A good method of ensuring that you reach the proper temperatures is to buy a decent candy thermometer for use in your soap making.

The thermometer should be used only for one particular type of soap and should be dedicated only to soap making. If you decide to experiment with soaps that have a variety of bases you will want to obtain a few thermometers since using the same thermometer for lye that you use for fat bases can throw off the results of your soap-making endeavor.

Thermometers can be found in most craft stores or in the cooking section of your grocery store. The thermometer you select does not need to be the most advanced or expensive model available. A simple, cost-effective thermometer will work just fine for these recipes.

Cooking Pot - You will need a glass or steel pot for heating and mixing.

You should have a dedicated mixing container for your soap making endeavors. While most of the ingredients in soap are safe, you would not want to eat out of the same pan you just used for boiling lye. You also want to be careful not to transfer foods, spices, and other cooking matter into your soap. These can irritate or worsen the conditions you are trying to treat.

It is important not to use aluminum or iron pots and pans when creating soap. The metal in these pots can react with the ingredients of the soap. A basic steel or enamel-coated pot works best and is often the most cost-effective purchase. You can find these in most retail chain stores.

Wooden Utensils - You will want to purchase a set of wooden utensils for soap making.

You should get a set of utensils that will be dedicated for use only with your product recipes. Again, these utensils should not be used for general cooking.

The type of utensils that have longer handles work well when making soap. You will need to stir deep into your cooking pots to ensure all the ingredients are well mixed and a longer handle makes it easier to stir and to prevent accidental contact between the ingredients and your hands.

Wooden utensils are heat resistant, will hold up better under some of the stronger ingredients you may choose to use, and will usually not cause an adverse reaction. You should not use metal utensils when making soap.

Gloves – You will want to use a pair of kitchen gloves to protect your hands from the ingredients used in soap making.

You will use the final product of your soap making process on your skin, but the core ingredients can cause irritation or even burns before they are diluted into the recipe. Using a pair of kitchen gloves is the best practice during your soap making. These will protect your hands from inadvertent splashing and prevent problems that will then need to be treated using a different recipe.

Soap Molds - You will need a mold or container to hold your completed soap during the hardening stage.

These recipes will often finish as a cake of soap. To achieve these perfectly formed cakes, you will need to use a mold. There are many molds available in specialty craft stores as well as at retail chain stores. Soap making has gained popularity in the last few years, making these products easier to find than ever before. You can find molds ranging from the very basic cake soap style to the more specialized styles that will suit your décor.

If you are using your soap yourself, you might not be as concerned with achieving the perfect appearance as you are with usefulness. You do not need to purchase specialized soap molds. Many items found in your house can be used as a mold.

You can use old baking pans such as muffin pans, cookie cutters, or bread pans as soap molds. You can even make your own mold out of old cardboard boxes. Almost any container that can withstand the heat of the liquid soap and will hold the liquid soap in place while it hardens will work as a mold.

Soap Making Dos!

When making soap, you must work in a well-ventilated area. Liquid and heated forms of some ingredients included in the soap making process can create fumes that may be harmful if inhaled.

Always wear gloves and other protective clothing when making soap since lye and other ingredients can burn or irritate the skin.

Always use COLD water when mixing lye solutions.

Pour the lye mixture into the fat mixture not the other way around.

Keep solvents like vinegar nearby to neutralize the effect of the ingredients if they should touch the skin.

Remember that lye is a poison and should always be kept in a safe place.

Only create heated soap mixtures when you can be sure that you will not be distracted. Some of the ingredients and the heat processes involved in soap making can be dangerous. In addition, the recipes included in this chapter require a fine attention to detail to ensure success in your soap-making endeavor.

Beeswax Soap

Beeswax soap is becoming more popular for all types of treatments and especially for the care of aging skin. The natural healing and antibacterial properties of beeswax make it a soap option with a wide range of uses. Beeswax also leaves a thin protective coating on the skin making it one of the better quality soaps for those with sensitive or dry skin.

Creating this soap is sometimes a bit more expensive than the other forms since beeswax can be more costly. Check with your health food stores or a beekeeping compound in your area to find the best price on beeswax.

The following recipe will make approximately 1 bar of soap. You can enlarge it if you want to make a bigger batch.

Heat 1/3 cup of your favorite vegetable-based oil.

Review the optional ingredient list to determine which oil will provide the most beneficial effect for your needs.

Add 4 tsp. grated beeswax to the oils and heat until melted. The mixture will be approximately 90 degrees.

While your oils are heating, dissolve 2 tsp. lye in 1/3 cup cold distilled water.

Remember to wear protective gloves and clothing when working with lye since lye can burn your skin.

Store your unused lye granules in a safe place since lye is a poison.

Remove your oil mixture from the heat and allow it to allow cool slightly until it reaches approximately 70 degrees.

While I do use additives that can prove beneficial for certain conditions, I typically do not add color or fragrance to any product designed for damaged or sensitive skin because additives can cause the irritation to worsen. If you prefer something other than the natural color or scent, you can add your favorite colorant, essential oils or herbs to the mixture.

Slowly pour the lye solution into the oil mixture.

Stir the mixture gently but well to ensure that all of the ingredients are blended.

If the soap mixture does not thicken within 30 minutes or if there is a greasy layer on the top of the mixture it may be too warm.

Set the container in a pan of cool water.

Continue stirring, making sure to stir the sides and bottom of the pan to ensure an even mix.

The mixture will become thicker taking on the consistency of syrup.

If the soap mixture is too lumpy, it may be too cold. If this occurs, reverse the above process.

Sit the mixture in a pan of warm water stirring until the lumps dissolve. You may need to replace the warm water more than once until the mixture is heated to the correct temperature for effective blending.

Remember that everyone's skin reacts differently. You should test the products on a less sensitive area before using them.

Pour the thickened mixture into your molds, cover, and keep it in a warm place for at least 2 days. This helps to keep the mixture from separating.

Once the soap has set, remove the finished soap from the molds and cut it into bars.

Place the soap in a dry area until you are ready to use it.

Castile Soap

A nice soap base alternative to traditional bars is castile soap. To be castile soap the mixture must contain at least 40% olive oil. You can purchase ready-made castile soap and then customize the mixture to suit your needs or you may create castile soap at home.

This soap is especially mild and gentle making it a good selection for aging, damaged or irritated skin. Castile soap is a versatile soap, you can even use the same castile soap products to wash your hair as you use for the rest of your body. You should test castile soap on a smaller area before using it in treatments for acne since the oils may cause extra irritation in some people.

The following recipe will yield the liquid equivalent of 1 bar of soap. You can increase the recipe if you want to make a larger batch.

Heat 1/3 cup of olive oil to approximately 90 degrees Fahrenheit.

While the oil is heating, dissolve 2 tsp. lye granules in 1/3 cup cold water.

Remember to wear protective gloves and clothing when working with lye since lye can burn your skin. Store your unused lye granules in a safe place because lye is a poison.

Remove your oil mixture from the heat and allow it to cool slightly until it reaches approximately 70 degrees.

While I do use additives that can prove beneficial for certain conditions, I typically do not add color or fragrance to any product designed for damaged or sensitive skin because additives can cause the irritation to worsen. If you prefer something other than the natural color or scent, you can add your favorite colorant, essential oils or herbs to the mixture.

Slowly pour the lye solution into the oil mixture.

Stir the mixture gently but well to ensure that all of the ingredients are well blended.

Allow the mixture to cool before placing it in a dispenser jar. If you want to convert liquid castile soap to a bar product, you will add a thickening agent and emulsifier and pour the finished mixture into molds as you would with any bar soap.

Remember that everyone's skin reacts differently. You should test the products on a less sensitive area before using them.

Coconut Oil Soap

Coconut oil is an excellent skin protecting agent and is one of the nicest natural foaming products that you can find to use in the soap making process

The following recipe will yield approximately 1 bar of soap. You can increase the recipe if you want a bigger batch.

Heat 3 teaspoons of coconut oil and ¼ cup vegetable-based oil on low heat to approximately 90 degrees Fahrenheit.

While the mixture is heating, dissolve 2 tsp. lye granules in 1/3 cup cold water.

Remember to wear protective gloves and clothing when working with lye since lye can burn your skin.

Store your unused lye granules in a safe place because lye is a poison.

Remove your oil mixture from the heat and allow it to cool slightly until t reaches approximately 70 degrees.

While I do use additives that can prove beneficial for certain conditions, I typically do not add color or fragrance to any product designed for damaged or sensitive skin because additives can cause the irritation to worsen. If you prefer something other than the natural color or scent, you can add your favorite colorant, essential oils or herbs to the mixture.

Slowly pour the lye solution into the oil mixture. Stir until the ingredients are well blended

If the soap mixture does not thicken within 30 minutes or there is a greasy layer on the top of the mixture it may be too warm.

Set the container in a pan of cool water. Stir the mixture, making certain that you stir the sides and bottom of the pan to ensure an even mix.

The mixture will become thicker taking on the consistency of syrup.

If the soap is lumpy, your mixture may be too cold. If this occurs, reverse the above process.

Sit the mixture in a pan of warm water stirring until the lumps dissolve. Depending on the consistency you may need to replace your warm water more than once until the mixture is heated to the correct temperature for effective blending.

Pour the thickened mixture into your molds, cover, and keep the mixture in a warm place for at least 2 days. This helps keep the soap from separating.

Remember that everyone's skin reacts differently. You should test the products on a less sensitive area before using them.

Tallow Based Soaps

Tallow has been used for generations in soap making and is considered one of the most common homemade soap products. Tallow soaps are made using the fat by-product trimmed from meat. You can collect clean fat as you cook. Simply trim off clean beef or pork fat before you cook your meat and save it, preferably in the freezer, until you are ready to make soap. Your local butcher or meat department will often provide you with free fat that is left when they trim their products.

One bar of soap will need approximately 1 cup of clean fat. You can increase the recipe if you want to create a bigger batch.

Place the fat in your soap-making pan and heat it until it is melted to an oil form.

Allow your mixture to cool to approximately 115 degrees Fahrenheit.

Add 1 tsp. of borax powder for each cup of melted fat. You do not have to add borax but it does give a better appearance and lather to your soap. If you add the borax, stir the powder into your tallow mixture until well blended.

While I do use additives that can prove beneficial for certain conditions, I typically do not add color or fragrance to any product designed for damaged or sensitive skin because additives can cause the irritation to worsen. If you prefer something other than the natural color or scent, you can add your favorite colorant, essential oils or herbs to the mixture.

While your tallow mixture is cooling to the desired temperature, you will need to create the lye solution. Again, remember to wear protective gloves and clothing when using lye because it can burn the skin.

Lye is a poison and unused amounts should be stored in a safe place.

Dissolve the lye granules in cool water.

You will use approximately 3 teaspoons of lye to ½ cup water for each bar of soap being created.

Once the lye granules are dissolved, you will slowly pour the lye mixture into the fat mixture.

Pour it in a slow steady stream while stirring the mixture.

You should not have the heat on the mixture at this time.

Stir the ingredients until thick syrup is formed. This should take approximately 10-20 minutes.

If the soap is not becoming thick after 30 minutes or has a greasy layer floating on the top, the mixture may be too warm.

Set the container in a pan of cool water.

Continue stirring, making sure to stir the sides and bottom of the pan to ensure an even mix.

If the soap is too lumpy, your mixture may be too cold.

If this occurs, reverse the above process.

Sit the mixture in a pan of warm water stirring until the lumps dissolve.

Depending on the consistency of the mixture, you may need to replace your warm water more than once until the soap is heated to the correct temperature.

Pour the thickened mixture into your molds, cover, and keep the mixture in a warm place for at least 2 days. This helps to keep the mixture from separating.

Once the soap has set, remove it from the molds and place it a dry area to age. Aging soap ensures a better quality final soap product. You should allow your tallow soap to age at least 2-3 weeks prior to use.

At times, you will find that your soap is lumpy or has separated during the aging process. If this occurs, do not throw out the failed soap.

Cut the flawed cakes of soap into small pieces. You can use an ordinary kitchen grater to cut the soap into smaller pieces.

Return the pieces to your soap-making pan and add approximately 1 cup of water for each cake of ground soap.

Dissolve the soap in the water over low heat. Stir the mixture occasionally to help distribute the heat.

When the lumps have disappeared and the mixture has formed a syrup, pour the soap into your favorite molds and follow the process for storage outlined earlier.

This will often cure the problem and provide you with a successful soap.

Remember that everyone's skin reacts differently. You should test the products on a less sensitive area before using them.

Glycerin Soap

One of the most common homemade cake soaps is a glycerin-based soap.

Glycerin is found naturally in many plants and is actually a by-product of the tallow soap making process. When making a fat and lye soap there is often a clear, thick liquid that floats on the top of the mixture. This is glycerin.

Glycerin soap is simply a basic soap that has extra glycerin added to the mixture. This soap is excellent for all skin types because it tends to be very mild. Glycerin is also a natural humectant that draws and retains moisture in your skin.

The following recipe will make approximately 1 bar of soap. You can increase the recipe if you want to make a bigger batch.

Heat 1/3 cup of your favorite vegetable-based oil to approximately 90 degrees.

Add 1 tsp. of borax powder for each bar of soap you are making. You do not need to add the borax powder but it will make a nicer final product. If you choose to add the borax powder to your soap, stir the oils and borax until they are well blended.

While your oils are heating, dissolve 2 tsp. lye in 1/3 cup cold water.

Remember to wear protective gloves and clothing when working with lye since it can burn your skin.

Store your unused lye granules in a safe place because lye is a poison.

Remove your oil mixture from the heat and allow it to cool to approximately 70 degrees.

While I do use additives that can prove beneficial for certain conditions, I typically do not add color or fragrance to any product designed for damaged or sensitive skin because additives can cause the irritation to worsen. If you prefer something other than the natural color or scent, you can add your favorite colorant, essential oils or herbs to the mixture.

Slowly pour the lye solution into the oil mixture.

Stir the mixture gently but mix well to ensure all of the ingredients are well blended.

When the ingredients are well blended, add 3 tsp. glycerin.

Continue stirring the mixture until the ingredients are well blended.

The mixture will take on the consistency of syrup.

If the soap mixture does not thicken within 30 minutes or if there is a greasy layer on the top of the mixture, it may be too warm.

Set the container in a pan of cool water.

Continue stirring, making sure to stir the sides and bottom of the pan to ensure an even mix.

If the soap mixture is too lumpy, your mixture may be too cold. If this occurs, reverse the above process.

Sit the mixture in a pan of warm water stirring until the lumps dissolve.

Depending on the consistency, you may need to replace your warm water more than once until the lumps dissolve.

Pour the thickened mixture into your molds, cover, and keep it in a warm place for at least 2 days. This helps to keep the mixture from separating.

Remember that everyone's skin reacts differently. You should test the products on a less sensitive area before using them.

Soap Variations

The soap recipes on the following pages provide some customizations that you can use with the soap base recipes. You can create your own soap using the recipes on the previous pages, purchase melt-and-pour soap from a natural product supplier, or buy mass-market soap to use as a base. You will then customize these bases with ingredients that suit your particular skin care needs.

The variations on these pages are some of my favorite soap customizations. The ingredient mixes will work well with any of the core soap bases described earlier. At times, there is a soap base that works exceptionally well for a particular customization. These are noted in the recipe as a suggestion.

Remember that everyone's skin reacts differently. You should test the products on a less sensitive area before using them.

Do not be afraid to replace an ingredient in the customization recipes if you feel there is a better alternative for your needs. Creating your own natural products is all about experimentation and customization. You should strive to use the ingredients that meet your particular needs in every recipe.

Soothing Oatmeal Soap

Perhaps my favorite soap modification is to add oatmeal to my soap base giving me a cleansing but soothing soap product. Oatmeal is gentle, soothing, and cleansing all at the same time. Oatmeal adds an exfoliating effect to the soap mixture while providing a soft, moist feel to the skin. Liquid based oatmeal soap is very versatile so a Castile base is an excellent choice. I also love adding these ingredients to my coconut oil soap.

1 tsp. Borax Powder

1/3 cup Jojoba Oil

1 tsp. Coconut Oil

Heat the borax and oil mixture to approximately 80 degrees in your soap-making pan, in the microwave, or using a double broiler. Remove the mixture from the heat. Mix the ingredients well and add

3 tsp. Glycerin

1/4 cup Oatmeal - Ground

Fragrance, Color, Emulsifier & Thickener as desired

While I do add herbs & oils that contain beneficial compounds, I typically do not add color or fragrance to any product designed for damaged skin because additives can cause the irritation to worsen. If you prefer something other than the natural color or scent, you can add your favorite colorant, essential oils or herbs to the mixture.

Pour the blended ingredients into your favorite soap base.

You may need to heat the mixture a second time before blending it with your soap base.

Continue stirring the mixture until the ingredients are well blended.

The mixture will become thicker as you stir. Pour the finished product into the soap molds of your choice and allow it to harden and age as directed by the soap base instructions.

Remember that everyone's skin reacts differently. You should test the products on a less sensitive area before using them.

Age Reversing Bar

This fantastic moisturizing soap also acts to counter aging, leaving the skin looking and feeling renewed. This recipe is used to make 1 bar of soap but can be increased to create a larger batch. This modification works especially well with coconut or beeswax bars.

1/3 cup Wheat Germ Oil

2 tbsp. Sea Buckthorn Oil

1 tsp. Glycerin

Heat the oils & glycerin to approximately 90 degrees in your soap-making pan, in the microwave, or using a double broiler.

Remove your oil mixture from the heat and allow it to cool to approximately 70 degrees.

3 tbsp. Powdered Seaweed

Add the powdered seaweed to the oils and stir the mixture until the ingredients are well blended.

While I do add herbs & oils that contain beneficial compounds, I typically do not add color or fragrance to any product designed for damaged skin because additives can cause the irritation to worsen. If you prefer something other than the natural color or scent, you can add your favorite colorant, essential oils or herbs to the mixture.

Pour the blended ingredients into your favorite soap base.

You may need to heat the mixture a second time before blending it with your soap base.

Continue stirring the mixture until the ingredients are well blended.

The mixture will become thicker as you stir. Pour the finished product into the soap molds of your choice and allow it to harden and age as directed by the soap base instructions.

Remember that everyone's skin reacts differently. You should test the products on a less sensitive area before using them.

Wonder Bars

These bars infuse moisture to the skin in a way that no other soap modification can. I absolutely love to use them during the winter months and they are an excellent choice for cleaning skin that has trouble retaining the moisture that is so important to keeping that youthful appearance. This modification works especially well in glycerin bars.

3 tbsp. Wheat Germ Oil

3 tbsp. Kukui Nut Oil

3 tbsp. Lavender Oil

1 tbsp. Honey

2 tbsp. Aloe Vera Gel

Create your soap base according to the instructions for the soap that you want t o use for this recipe. I prefer glycerin soap as a base for this recipe.

Cool the soap base to approximately 70 degrees and add the modification ingredients. Stir until the ingredients are well blended in your soap base.

While I do add herbs & oils that contain beneficial compounds, I typically do not add color or fragrance to any product designed for damaged skin because additives can cause the irritation to worsen. If you prefer something other than the natural color or scent, you can add your favorite colorant, essential oils or herbs to the mixture.

Pour the blended ingredients into your favorite soap base.

Continue stirring the mixture until the ingredients are well blended.

The mixture will become thicker as you stir. Pour the finished product into the soap molds of your choice and allow it to harden and age as directed by the soap base instructions.

Remember that everyone's skin reacts differently. You should test the products on a less sensitive area before using them.

Hydrating Apple Soap

Hydration is essential for beautiful, healthy skin and this soap not only infuses the skin with moisture it also helps to sooth irritation. This is a great choice when you have itchy, irritated, or dried skin. This modification works very well with a beeswax soap base. The juice helps to attract moisture, the beeswax protects from irritants, and the chlorophyll speeds healing.

Create the soap base of your choice according to the instructions. Add

2 tbsp. Apple Juice

1 tsp. Liquid Chlorophyll

The mixture will have a delicate apple scent and a lovely green color. If you desire a different color or fragrance, you may add food coloring or the desired essential oils to the mixture.

While I do add herbs & oils that contain beneficial compounds, I typically do not add color or fragrance to any product designed for damaged skin because additives can cause the irritation to worsen.

The mixture will become thicker as you stir. Pour the finished product into the soap molds of your choice and allow it to harden and age as directed by the soap base instructions.

Remember that everyone's skin reacts differently. You should test the products on a less sensitive area before using them.

Exfoliating Bars

This soap is an excellent choice when you want a soap that will hydrate and exfoliate all in one. It helps to remove dead skin cells, oils, and dirt while leaving the skin looking and feeling clean & refreshed. You will be amazed at how moist and clear you skin looks after using this soap.

1 tsp Borax Powder

1/3 cup Hazelnut Oil

1 tsp. Coconut Oil

2 tsp. Grated Beeswax

Melt the beeswax until it reaches around 90 degrees Fahrenheit and has a liquid appearance. Remove the beeswax from the heat and add the borax powder & oil to the base. Borax in not a necessary ingredient for this recipe but it can improve the appearance and performance of your soap.

Add

2 tsp. Lye Granules

1/3 cup Cold Distilled Water

1/8 cup Carrot Juice

Stir the mixture until the ingredients are well blended.

The mixture will have an orange appearance. If you desire a specific color or fragrance for your soap, you may add your favorite food coloring or essential oils.

While I do add herbs & oils that contain beneficial compounds, I typically do not add color or fragrance to any product designed for damaged skin because additives can cause the irritation to worsen.

Pour the soap solution of your choice into the base. You can simply increase the amount of beeswax too instead of adding a soap base. This will help the mixture to solidify.

When the ingredients are well blended, add the remaining ingredients.

3 tsp. Glycerin

1 Orange Peel grated medium fine

Continue stirring the mixture until well blended. The mixture will become thicker taking on the consistency of syrup.

The mixture will become thicker as you stir. Pour the finished product into the soap molds of your choice and allow it to harden and age as directed by the soap base instructions.

Remember that everyone's skin reacts differently. You should test the products on a less sensitive area before using them.

Skin Lightening Bars

One of the hardest issues to remedy is the darkening that sometimes occurs with aging skin. This pigmentation includes age spots, seborrhea scarring, freckles, or a darker cast to an entire area of skin. This beeswax soap modification is wonderful for hydrating and soothing aged skin while helping to lighten the natural darkening that can occur as skin ages.

1/4 cup Peanut Oil

2 tbsp. Grated Beeswax

1 tbsp. Honey

Heat the mixture for approximately 25 seconds on medium heat in the microwave or to approximately 90 degrees in a double broiler. The melted ingredients will take on a syrupy consistency.

Remove your oil mixture from the heat and allow it to cool to approximately 70 degrees. Add

2 tbsp. Bitter Damson - Powdered

1/2 tsp. Andiroba Oil

1/2 tsp. Kukui Nut Oil

While I do add herbs & oils that contain beneficial compounds, I typically do not add color or fragrance to any product designed for damaged skin because additives can cause the irritation to worsen. If you prefer something other than the natural color or scent, you can add your favorite colorant, essential oils or herbs to the mixture.

Pour the soap solution of your choice into the oil mixture and blend well.

The mixture will become thicker as you stir. Pour the finished product into the soap molds of your choice and allow it to harden and age as directed by the soap base instructions.

Remember that everyone's skin reacts differently. You should test the products on a less sensitive area before using them.

Skin Brightening Bars

Reducing the appearance of dark pigmentation is an important step to combating aging skin. Another important step is to brighten & tone the skin. These bars help to brighten the skin while adding a nice toned, hydrated look.

1/4 cup Coconut Oil

2 tbsp. Grated Beeswax

1 tbsp. Grape Seed Oil

Heat the mixture for approximately 25 seconds on medium heat in the microwave or to approximately 90 degrees in a double broiler. The melted ingredients will take on a syrupy consistency.

Remove your oil mixture from the heat and allow it to cool to approximately 70 degrees.   Add

2 tbsp. Powdered Basil

1/2 tsp. Geranium Oil

1/2 tsp. Lemon Oil

While I do add herbs & oils that contain beneficial compounds, I typically do not add color or fragrance to any product designed for damaged skin because additives can cause the irritation to worsen. If you prefer something other than the natural color or scent, you can add your favorite colorant, essential oils or herbs to the mixture.

Pour the soap solution of your choice into the oil mixture and blend well.

The mixture will become thicker as you stir. Pour the finished product into the soap molds of your choice and allow it to harden and age as directed by the soap base instructions.

Remember that everyone's skin reacts differently. You should test the products on a less sensitive area before using them.

Toning Bars

This is an amazing skin-toning recipe that helps to infuse moisture and reduce the appearance of oversized pores while gently toning and tightening the skin.

1/4 cup Almond Oil

2 tbsp. Grated Beeswax

1 tbsp. Honey

Heat the mixture for approximately 25 seconds on medium heat in the microwave or to approximately 90 degrees in a double broiler. The melted ingredients will take on a syrupy consistency.

Remove your oil mixture from the heat and allow it to cool to approximately 70 degrees. Add

2 tbsp. Powdered Basil

2 tsp. Carob Powder

1 tsp. Borax Powder

1 tsp. Cypress Oil

2 tsp. Fennel Oil

Stir the mixture until the ingredients are well blended.

While I do add herbs & oils that contain beneficial compounds, I typically do not add color or fragrance to any product designed for damaged skin because additives can cause the irritation to worsen. If you prefer something other than the natural color or scent, you can add your favorite colorant, essential oils or herbs to the mixture.

Pour the soap solution of your choice into the oil mixture and blend well.

The mixture will become thicker as you stir. Pour the finished product into the soap molds of your choice and allow it to harden and age as directed by the soap base instructions.

Remember that everyone's skin reacts differently. You should test the products on a less sensitive area before using them.

Collagen Building Bars

One of the biggest factors contributing to the aged appearance of skin is a loss of collagen. Research has illustrated that certain compounds in plant products actually help stimulate collagen production. These bars contain my favorite blend of collagen stimulating and regenerative ingredients.

1/4 cup Sunflower Oil

2 tbsp. Grated Beeswax

2 tbsp.   Grape Seed Oil

Heat the mixture for approximately 25 seconds on medium heat in the microwave or to approximately 90 degrees in a double broiler. The melted ingredients will take on a syrupy consistency.

Remove your oil mixture from the heat and allow it to cool to approximately 70 degrees. Add

2 tbsp. Gotu Kola

1/2 tsp. Myrrh Oil

1/2 tsp. Immortelle

While I do add herbs & oils that contain beneficial compounds, I typically do not add color or fragrance to any product designed for damaged skin because additives can cause the irritation to worsen. If you prefer something other than the natural color or scent, you can add your favorite colorant. essential oils or herbs to the mixture.

Pour the soap solution of your choice into the oil mixture and blend well.

The mixture will become thicker as you stir. Pour the finished product into the soap molds of your choice and allow it to harden and age as directed by the soap base instructions.

Remember that everyone's skin reacts differently. You should test the products on a less sensitive area before using them.

Silkening Bars

Sometimes, we need to concentrate on pampering our skin, not just reducing the appearance of aging. This soap not only helps to tighten the skin, it adds a lovely, supple feeling. I love to use these bars whenever my skin is healthy overall and I can spend some time pampering.

1/4 cup Jojoba Oil

4 tsp. Grated Beeswax

Heat the mixture for approximately 25 seconds on medium heat in the microwave or to approximately 90 degrees in a double broiler. The melted ingredients will take on a syrupy consistency.

Remove your oil mixture from the heat and allow it to cool to approximately 70 degrees. Add

2 tbsp. Evening Primrose Oil

2 tbsp. Glycerin

3 tbsp. Pomegranate Oils

Stir the mixture until all of the ingredients are well blended.

While I do add herbs & oils that contain beneficial compounds, I typically do not add color or fragrance to any product designed for damaged skin because additives can cause the irritation to worsen. If you prefer something other than the natural color or scent, you can add your favorite colorant, essential oils or herbs to the mixture.

Pour the soap solution of your choice into the oil mixture and blend well.

The mixture will become thicker as you stir. Pour the finished product into the soap molds of your choice and allow it to harden and age as directed by the soap base instructions.

Remember that everyone's skin reacts differently. You should test the products on a less sensitive area before using them.

Bedtime Bars

This is a favorite of mine at night before bed. The natural aroma of lavender and chamomile provide a relaxing benefit minimizing stress while the soap itself softens and hydrates the skin, reducing puffiness. I typically follow this treatment with a hydrating moisturizer and wake with beautiful, moisturized skin.

1 tsp. Chamomile Leaves

1 tsp. Basil

1/4 cup Water

Heat the Water to the boiling point and pour it over the leaves. Do not immerse the leaves in boiling Water since this might minimize the beneficial compounds contained in the plant parts. Allow the leaves and Water to soak overnight. The mixture should form a very strong tea. You can stain the plant parts from the mixture or leave them in to give added power to the finished soap.

3 tbsp. Grated Beeswax

Heat the beeswax for approximately 25 seconds on medium heat in the microwave or to approximately 90 degrees in a double broiler. The melted ingredients will take on a syrupy consistency. Remove mixture from the heat and allow it to cool to approximately 70 degrees.

1 tsp. Borax Powder

Dissolve the borax powder in the wax base. Borax in not a necessary ingredient for this recipe but it can improve the appearance and performance of your soap.

When the mixture is well blended, add the remaining ingredients.

1 tbsp. Coconut Oil

3 tbsp. Jojoba Oil

3 tsp. Lavender Oil

1 tsp. Lemon Juice

3 tsp. Glycerin

While I do add herbs & oils that contain beneficial compounds, I typically do not add color or fragrance to any product designed for damaged skin because additives can cause the irritation to worsen. If you prefer something other than the natural color or scent, you can add your favorite colorant, essential oils or herbs to the mixture.

Pour the soap solution of your choice into the oil mixture and blend well.

The mixture will become thicker as you stir. Pour the finished product into the soap molds of your choice and allow it to harden and age as directed by the soap base instructions.

Remember that everyone's skin reacts differently. You should test the products on a less sensitive area before using them.

Soft Soaps & Cleansers

Every inch of your skin is important and deserves to be treated with care but certain areas require specialized attention. Soft soaps and cleansers are a preferred choice for some people, especially when treating facial skin. Soft cleansers help to remove the dirt, oils, bacteria, and other toxins that can increase the processes of environmental aging without aggravating sensitive skin.

Cleansing is one of the best places that you can spend time experimenting and customizing the recipes to suit your needs. The better customized your cleansing regimen is to your particular skin type, lifestyle, and needs the better your overall appearance will be.

You may need to use different cleansers on different parts of your skin. The face & neck area tends to need different treatments and preventatives than other skin like elbows & knees. You should consider the goal of the treatment, sensitivity of the areas being treated, and personal application preferences before selecting recipes to try.

Regardless of the recipes you choose to try it is always recommended that you test sample the products on a sensitive area such as your wrist to ensure that you do not have unexpected reactions before applying them to your skin. This is not a fail proof method of ensuring that the products are correct for you but it can often provide a warning of a negative reaction.

Gentle Foaming Scrub

Foaming washes are one of my favorite types of facial cleansers. The foaming action helps to clean the skin and makes application a breeze. This is a favorite cleaner of mine since it is gentle enough for year round use and the natural ingredients help to tighten my skin, combat environmental aging, and improve the overall look and texture of my skin.

3 tbsp. Coconut Oil

1 tbsp. Apricot Kernel Oil

1 tbsp. Palmarosa Oil

1 tsp. Fennel Oil

Emulsifier & Thickener as desired

Gently stir the oils until they are well blended. Do not whip this recipe since the coconut oil will foam. If the coconut oil is too solid for blending, you can warm it between the palms of your hand to soften it.

This recipe has a delicate, sweet smell but if you desire a specific color or fragrance, you may add your favorite colorant or essential oils or herbs to the mixture.

While I do add herbs & oils that contain beneficial compounds, I typically do not add color or fragrance to any product designed for damaged skin because additives can cause the irritation to worsen.

Spoon mixture into a clean container and seal it tightly.

To use, place a small amount in the palm of your hand, mix with water, and scrub your face with a gentle upward motion. This is a soap mixture so always rinse your skin thoroughly when done washing.

Remember that everyone's skin reacts differently. You should test the products on a less sensitive area before using them.

Toning Daily Cleanser

This recipe makes a nice, gentle cleanser that is gentle enough for daily use. It helps to combat the most common causes of environmental aging while toning & softening the skin.

1/2 cup Aloe Vera Gel

1 tbsp. Carob Powder

1 tbsp. Hazelnut Oil

3 tbsp. Witch Hazel

1/4 tsp. Geranium Oil

Emulsifier & Thickener as desired

Blend the ingredients in a blender or food processor until they are smooth.

While I do add herbs & oils that contain beneficial compounds, I typically do not add color or fragrance to any product designed for damaged skin because additives can cause the irritation to worsen.

Spoon mixture into a clean container and seal it tightly.

To use, place a small amount in the palm of your hand, mix with water, and scrub your face with a gentle upward motion. This is a soap mixture so always rinse your skin thoroughly when done washing.

Remember that everyone's skin reacts differently. You should test the products on a less sensitive area before using them.

Daily Cleanser with Toning Agents

This recipe visibly reduces the appearance of pores while helping to combat the speed of the aging processes. It also provides a balm that helps heal damaged skin while giving a light toning action. I modify the recipe by adding ingredients from the alternate ingredient list throughout the year to get the most beneficial results for each season. You can use this cleanser alone or add additional ingredients from the list to ensure the best results for your skin type.

2 tbsp. Borage Seed Oil

3 tsp. Honey

1/4 cup Rosewater

1 tsp. Borax Powder

1 tbsp. Fennel Oil

Emulsifier & Thickener as desired

Gently stir the ingredients until they are well blended.

While I do add herbs & oils that contain beneficial compounds, I typically do not add color or fragrance to any product designed for damaged skin because additives can cause the irritation to worsen. If you prefer something other than the natural color or scent, you can add your favorite colorant, essential oils or herbs to the mixture.

Store the mixture in a tightly sealed container.

To use, massage a small amount into your skin using an upward motion. Let the mixture sit on the skin for 30 – 60 seconds before rinsing. This is a soap mixture so always rinse your skin thoroughly when done washing.

Remember that everyone's skin reacts differently. You should test the products on a less sensitive area before using them.

Daily Moisture Infusing Cleanser

This light cleanser combines moisture-infusing ingredients with a very gentle cleansing action. It makes a good selection for preventative daily cleansing especially for those who have very dry skin.

1/2 cup Castile Soap

1/8 cup Rose Hip Oil

1 tbsp. Palmarosa Oil

1 tbsp. Grape Seed Oil

Mix all of the ingredients until they are well blended.

While I do add herbs & oils that contain beneficial compounds, I typically do not add color or fragrance to any product designed for damaged skin because additives can cause the irritation to worsen. If you prefer something other than the natural color or scent, you can add your favorite colorant, essential oils or herbs to the mixture.

Store the mixture in a tightly sealed container.

To use, massage a small amount into your skin using an upward motion.

Let the mixture sit on the skin for 30 – 60 seconds before rinsing.

This is a soap mixture so always rinse your skin thoroughly when done washing.

Remember that everyone's skin reacts differently. You should test the products on a less sensitive area before using them.

Soothing Wash

Nighttime is one of the best times to pamper yourself and your skin. This recipe makes a wonderful nighttime cleanser. The scent and compounds in the lavender give a soothing effect to both your skin and your mind. The other ingredients help to tighten, tone, and heal the skin. I also use this wash as a bath additive when I need a relaxing bath to help prepare for bed or a full body cleanser.

1/4 tsp. Tincture of Benzoin

1 tbsp. Distilled Water

3 tbsp. Witch Hazel

3-4 drops Lavender Oil

1 tsp. Glycerin

3 tbsp. Aloe Vera Gel

Gently combine all of the ingredients until they well blended.

While I do add herbs & oils that contain beneficial compounds, I typically do not add color or fragrance to any product designed for damaged skin because additives can cause the irritation to worsen. If you prefer something other than the natural color or scent, you can add your favorite colorant, essential oils or herbs to the mixture.

Store the mixture in a tightly sealed container.

To use, massage a small amount into your skin using an upward motion. Let the mixture sit on the skin for 30 – 60 seconds before rinsing. This is a soap mixture so always rinse your skin thoroughly when done washing.

Remember that everyone's skin reacts differently. You should test the products on a less sensitive area before using them.

Brightening Scrub

This foaming wash combines a gentle cleansing agent with brightening ingredients, and an easy application. It is my first choice for a quick cleanser especially when I am trying to combat dull looking skin.

3 tbsp. Coconut Oil

1 tsp. Angelica Oil

1 tsp Geranium Oil

3 tbsp. Witch Hazel

1/4 tsp. Tincture of Benzoin

1 crushed Vitamin C Tablet

Dissolve the Vitamin C powder in the witch hazel mixture.

Gently stir the mixture until the remaining ingredients are blended into the base.

The mixture will foam if it is stirred too vigorously.

While I do add herbs & oils that contain beneficial compounds, I typically do not add color or fragrance to any product designed for damaged skin because additives can cause the irritation to worsen. If you prefer something other than the natural color or scent, you can add your favorite colorant, essential oils or herbs to the mixture.

Store the mixture in a tightly sealed container.

To use, massage a small amount into your skin using an upward motion. Let the mixture sit on the skin for 30 – 60 seconds before rinsing. This is a soap mixture so always rinse your skin thoroughly when done washing.

Remember that everyone's skin reacts differently. You should test the products on a less sensitive area before using them.

Collagen Building Balm

I like to use a collagen building soap on every part of my body. Everything from deep scarring after a blemish to skin sagging & wrinkling relates to the lack of collagen in the skin. This nice foaming cleanser blends some of my favorite collagen building & skin regenerating ingredients into a healing cleansing agent.

2 tbsp. Borax Powder

1/4 cup Witch Hazel

1/4 cup Aloe Vera Gel

1 tbsp. Vitamin E Oil

2 tbsp. Myrrh Oil

1 tbsp. Baobab Oil

Dissolve borax powder in the witch hazel base. Add the remaining ingredients and blend well.

While I do add herbs & oils that contain beneficial compounds, I typically do not add color or fragrance to any product designed for damaged skin because additives can cause the irritation to worsen. If you prefer something other than the natural color or scent, you can add your favorite colorant, essential oils or herbs to the mixture.

Pour the finished mixture into clean container and seal tightly.

To use, pour small amount in the palm of your hand or apply it with a gentle upward motion. Allow the mixture to sit on your skin for 30-60 seconds before rinsing. This is also an excellent cleanser to add to your favorite scrubbing sacks. This is a soap mixture so always rinse your skin thoroughly when done washing.

Remember that everyone's skin reacts differently. You should test the products on a less sensitive area before using them.

Seborrhea Cleanser

This cleanser works well at combating seborrhea, which is a very common problem affecting aging skin. The yogurt infuses moisture into the skin while the lemon juice & sweet gale oils help to restore the skins natural acid levels minimizing seborrhea while brightening the complexion.

1/2 cup Unflavored Yogurt

1 tbsp. Sweet Gale Oil

2 tsp. Lemon Juice

Emulsifier & Thickener as desired

Mix the ingredients in a food processor or stir by hand until they are well blended.

While I do add herbs & oils that contain beneficial compounds, I typically do not add color or fragrance to any product designed for damaged skin because additives can cause the irritation to worsen. If you prefer something other than the natural color or scent, you can add your favorite colorant, essential oils or herbs to the mixture.

Store the finished mixture in a tightly sealed container. A pump bottles work well with this base. To use, pump a pea sized drop into the palm of your hand and massage it into your skin using an upward motion. Allow the cleanser to sit on your skin for 30-60 seconds before rinsing. This is a soap mixture so always rinse your skin thoroughly when done washing.

Remember that everyone's skin reacts differently. You should test the products on a less sensitive area before using them.

Alternative Soap for Seborrhea

This great moisturizing cleanser helps to reduce the severity of seborrhea without adding irritants that may aggravate the skin. It works especially well for people whose skin is sensitive.

1/4 cup Aloe Vera Gel

1 tsp. Borax Powder

3 tbsp. Distilled Water

1/2 tsp. Damask Rose

1/2 tsp. Sweet Gale

Emulsifier & Thickener as desired

Dissolve the borax powder in the water.

Mix with the remaining ingredients in a food processor or stir them by hand until a creamy gel has formed.

While I do add herbs & oils that contain beneficial compounds, I typically do not add color or fragrance to any product designed for damaged skin because additives can cause the irritation to worsen. If you prefer something other than the natural color or scent, you can add your favorite colorant, essential oils, or herbs to the mixture.

Store the finished mixture in a tightly sealed container. A pump bottles work well with this base. To use, pump a pea sized drop into the palm of your hand and massage it into your skin using an upward motion. Allow the cleanser to sit on your skin for 30-60 seconds before rinsing. This is a soap mixture so always rinse your skin thoroughly when done washing.

Remember that everyone's skin reacts differently. You should test the products on a less sensitive area before using them.

Age Spot Reduction Gel

Age spots, freckles, and even acne scars can contribute to the aged appearance of the skin. This wonderful gel helps to reduce those spots while tightening and toning the skin.

2 tbsp. Aloeswood Powder

2 tsp. Kukui Nut Oil

2 tsp. Immortelle

1/4 cup Distilled Water

1/4 cup Aloe Vera Gel

2 tbsp. Glycerin

2 tbsp. Papaya Milk

Emulsifier & Thickener as desired

Heat the water to a low simmer and add the powders. Continue to heat the mixture for about 2 minutes at a low simmer, stirring frequently until it thickens. If mixture becomes thicker than desired, you may add additional water until you obtain the consistency you prefer.

Remove the mixture from the heat and add the remaining ingredients. Stir the cleanser gently until all of the ingredients are well blended.

While I do add herbs & oils that contain beneficial compounds, I typically do not add color or fragrance to any product designed for damaged skin because additives can cause the irritation to worsen. If you prefer something other than the natural color or scent, you can add your favorite colorant, essential oils, or herbs to the mixture.

Store the finished mixture in a tightly sealed container. A pump bottle works well with this base. To use, pump a pea sized drop into the palm of your hand and massage it into your skin using an upward motion. Allow the cleanser to sit on your skin for 30-60 seconds before rinsing. This is a soap mixture so always rinse your skin thoroughly when done washing.

Remember that everyone's skin reacts differently. You should test the products on a less sensitive area before using them.

Healing Cleanser

This is an excellent cleansing gel for both the face and the body. We use it whenever our skin is overstressed, irritated, or we just need a bit of skin help. The arrowroot powder helps to condition the skin aiding it in retaining moisture while promoting healing. The glycerin attracts moisture, promoting repair of the damage and helping to give a hydrated, supple look to the skin.

2 cups Distilled Water

2 tbsp. Abscess Root

1 tbsp. Arrowroot Powder

1 tbsp. Apple Cider Vinegar

2 tbsp. Glycerin

Emulsifier & Thickener as desired

Heat the water to a light boil. Remove the water from the heat and add the abscess root. Allow the mixture to steep for 4-6 hours until a dark tea has formed. Strain the plant parts from the liquid. The fluid will become the base for your recipe.

Re-heat the water until it is warm but not hot and add the powders. Stir the mixture until the powders are dissolved and the mixture begins to thicken. If mixture becomes thicker than desired, you may add additional water until you obtain the consistency you prefer.

Add the remaining ingredients and stir the cleanser gently until it is well blended.

While I do add herbs & oils that contain beneficial compounds, I typically do not add color or fragrance to any product designed for damaged skin because additives can cause the irritation to worsen. If you prefer something other than the natural color or scent, you can add your favorite colorant, essential oils, or herbs to the mixture.

Store the finished mixture in a tightly sealed container. A pump bottle works well with this base. To use, pump a pea sized drop into the palm of your hand and massage it into your skin using an upward motion. Allow the cleanser to sit on your skin for 30-60 seconds before rinsing. This is a soap mixture so always rinse your skin thoroughly when done washing.

Remember that everyone's skin reacts differently. You should test the products on a less sensitive area before using them.

Daily Damage Control Cleanser

This cleanser is mildly astringent helping to reduce the size of pores and give the skin a clean, fresh look. The addition of juice and aloe vera gel helps to combat dryness and repair damage. The ingredients also aid in the prevention of new fine lines & wrinkles.

1 tsp. Borax powder

1/4 cup Distilled Water

Heat the water to a low simmer and add the powders. Continue to heat the mixture for about 2 minutes at a low simmer, stirring frequently.

Remove the mixture from the heat and add the remaining ingredients.

2 tbsp Apple juice

2 tsp. Aloe Vera Gel

1 tsp. Carrot Oil

1 tsp. Geranium

Emulsifier & Thickener as desired

Stir the cleanser gently until all of the ingredients are well blended.

This mixture will be slightly looser than the others so you may wish to add a thickening agent for easier application.

This recipe has a lovely sweet smell and a pretty color but if you desire a specific color or fragrance, you may add your favorite colorant or essential oils or herbs to the mixture.

While I do add herbs & oils that contain beneficial compounds, I typically do not add color or fragrance to any product designed for damaged skin because additives can cause the irritation to worsen.

Store the finished mixture in a tightly sealed container. A pump bottle works well with this base. To use, pump a pea sized drop into the palm of your hand and massage it into your skin using an upward motion. Allow the cleanser to sit on your skin for 30-60 seconds before rinsing. This is a soap mixture so always rinse your skin thoroughly when done washing.

Remember that everyone's skin reacts differently. You should test the products on a less sensitive area before using them.

Beauty Milk Cleanser

Milk has long been considered a beauty treatment. This milk cleanser is excellent for infusing the skin with moisture while aiding in the restoration of the natural PH. The wash helps to improve both the texture and appearance of the skin.

1/4 cup Dry Milk Powder

2 tbsp. Rosewater

2 tbsp. Borage Seed Oil

2 tsp. Strawberry Leaf Powder

Emulsifier & Thickener as desired

Mix the ingredients in a food processor or stir by hand until they form a thick paste.

If the finished mixture is too thick, you may add a few drops of distilled water or rose water until you obtain the consistency you prefer.

While I do add herbs & oils that contain beneficial compounds, I typically do not add color or fragrance to any product designed for damaged skin because additives can cause the irritation to worsen. If you prefer something other than the natural color or scent, you can add your favorite colorant, essential oils, or herbs to the mixture.

This mixture will be very thick. Spoon it into a clean container with a tight fitting lid. To use, scoop a pea sized amount into the palm of your hand, mix in a few drops of water, and massage it into your skin using an upward motion. Allow the cleanser to sit on your skin for 30-60 seconds before rinsing. This is a soap mixture so always rinse your skin thoroughly when done washing.

Remember that everyone's skin reacts differently. You should test the products on a less sensitive area before using them.

Sweet Radiance Cleanser

Youthful skin has a well-hydrated, radiant glow. This cleanser helps to bring some of that refreshed appearance back to aging skin. Hydration from the inside and the outside is critical to helping your skin regain and retain that radiant glow.

2 tbsp. Plain Yogurt

1 tsp. Honey

1 tbsp. Geranium Oil

1 tbsp. Fennel Oil

1 tbsp. Rosewater (you may use Witch Hazel if desired)

Emulsifier & Thickener as desired

Place all of the ingredients in a blender and mix well.

While I do add herbs & oils that contain beneficial compounds, I typically do not add color or fragrance to any product designed for damaged skin because additives can cause the irritation to worsen. This cleanser has a beautiful light fragrance of its own, but if you desire a specific color or fragrance, you may add your favorite colorant or essential oils or herbs to the mixture.

Spoon the mixture into a clean container and seal it tightly.

Refrigeration may lengthen the shelf life of the product. This recipe makes one or two applications. If you choose to enlarge the recipe, refrigeration is necessary.

To use, place a small amount of the paste in the palm of your hand and apply to your skin in an upward motion. Allow the cleanser to sit on the 30-60 seconds before rinsing. This is a soap mixture so always rinse your skin thoroughly when done washing.

Remember that everyone's skin reacts differently. You should test the products on a less sensitive area before using them.

Skin Smoothing Cleanser

This is an excellent cleaner that I like to use in the winter months when my skin can begin to look dull and blotchy. It helps to tighten and tone my skin while improving the texture. It also helps to prevent redness, dry patches, and speed healing of any skin irritation.

1/2 cup Aloe Vera Gel

1 tbsp. Powdered Milk

1/4 cup Witch Hazel

2 tbsp. Peanut Oil

1 tbsp. Elderberry

Emulsifier & Thickener as desired

Mix all of the ingredients in a blender until a gel has formed.

The mixture will be looser and works very well in a pump. You may want to consider adding a beneficial thickening agent like Acacia Powder to the mixture for easier application.

While I do add herbs & oils that contain beneficial compounds, I typically do not add color or fragrance to any product designed for damaged skin because additives can cause the irritation to worsen. If you prefer something other than the natural color or scent, you can add your favorite colorant, essential oils, or herbs to the mixture.

To use apply a small amount to your skin massaging in an upward motion. Allow the cleanser to sit on the skin for 30-60 seconds before rinsing. This is a soap mixture so always rinse your skin thoroughly when done washing.

Remember that everyone's skin reacts differently. You should test the products on a less sensitive area before using them.

Soothing Wash

This is one of the more soothing skin washes. It works best when skin irritation is the most severe. It helps to hydrate while easing the inflammation.

1 tbsp. Marshmallow Root

1 cup Warm Water

Marshmallow Root tends to respond best as a cold infusion. The water should be warm, not hot when you add the root. Place the mixture in a cool place and allow the root to steep for up to 24 hours. Strain the marshmallow root from the liquid. The liquid should be a bit thicker than a regular tea. Add

3 tsp. Aloe Vera Gel

1 tsp. Sandalwood Oil

1 tsp. Geranium Oil

Emulsifier & Thickener as desired

Stir the remaining ingredients into the marshmallow root liquid until they are well blended.

While I do add herbs & oils that contain beneficial compounds, I typically do not add color or fragrance to any product designed for damaged skin because additives can cause the irritation to worsen. If you prefer something other than the natural color or scent, you can add your favorite colorant, essential oils, or herbs to the mixture.

Pour the mixture into a clean, dry bottle with a tight fitting lid.

The mixture will separate if it is left standing so shake the cleanser well before each use.

Apply to the skin with a gentle upward motion. Allow the cleanser to sit on the skin for 30-60 seconds before rinsing. This is a soap mixture so always rinse your skin thoroughly when done washing.

Remember that everyone's skin reacts differently. You should test the products on a less sensitive area before using them.

Exfoliating Scrubs

Sometimes dirt, oils, and dead skin cells build up on the skin. An exfoliating cleanser helps remove the build up and condition the skin in preparation for other treatments. Exfoliation is the act of lightly abrading the skin to help remove dead skin cells and reveal new, healthy skin cells.

Exfoliation is an important step toward obtaining the healthy, glowing skin you desire. Exfoliation not only removes dead cells and impurities, but the process of removing these cells actually allows your skin to retain moisture.

These specialized products may be used in place of or in addition to your regular cleanser.

Abrasive cleansers can irritate the skin. You should always test any new product before using it to determine exactly how your skin will react. If your test patch tolerates the scrub well, try using it a few times a week and see how much better your daily treatments perform.

Grain Scrubs

I love to have a handful of grains available to scrub my face and body every time I shower. I use these scrubs before my soap to remove any surface dirt and oils and to exfoliate my skin in preparation for the remaining treatments in my daily regimen.

You can use many different cleansing grains. The easiest to find and the ones I have found the most effective are:

Uncooked Oatmeal

Cornmeal

Wheat Germ

You may combine these grains or use them individually for great results. Just combine the selected grains with warm distilled water to form a paste. Massage the mixture into your skin with gentle circular motions. Rinse your skin well and follow the treatment with your favorite daily care products.

You can also blend the grains with a cold cream or soap for a foaming action.

Sometimes the loose grains are messy so I use a bag for application. You can make a scrubbing bag out of almost any material but a looser fabric works best. I prefer using muslin cloth cut to size but gauze or cheesecloth squares work well. Mix your favorite grains, grated soap, and oils together in a bowl and spoon the mixture onto your chosen cloth. Tie the cloth closed and you have an excellent rubbing bag for your bath.

While I do add herbs & oils that contain beneficial compounds, I typically do not add color or fragrance to any product designed for damaged skin because additives can cause the irritation to worsen. If you prefer something other than the natural color or scent, you can add your favorite colorant, essential oils, or herbs to the mixture.

Remember that everyone's skin reacts differently. You should test the products on a less sensitive area before using them.

Fruit Scrubs

Fruit pits & peels contain many of the same benefits and oils as the fruit itself and of the oils extracted from the fruit. I like to have a stronger exfoliation scrub available for more focused care of the rougher patches of my skin such as elbows, knees and feet.

There are many types of fruit pits available for you to use in your scrubs. You can choose any of the basic fruit pits listed below or experiment with other fruits to see what might work best for your particular needs.

There are many different fruit pits available in the scrubs sold at your local stores. You can also make your own single or blended fruit pit exfoliation product. You can choose any of the basic fruit pits listed below or experiment with other fruits to see what might work best for your particular needs.

Avocado Pit is very rich in oils that provide exceptional skin softening and conditioning with a more abrasive rubbing action than some other options.

Apricot Kernel contains oils that may be the easiest fruit oil for the skin to absorb. These oils are rich in Vitamin A that is vital for healthy, glowing skin.

Peach Pit is rich in conditioning oils that will aid in keeping skin soft and supple while acting as mild humectant to attract additional moisture to the surface of the skin.

To create a scrub, remove the hard shell from the outside of the pit or seed. Inside the hard shell will be an oil rich nut like product. Grind the nut to the desired consistency.

The larger the finished pieces the more intense the abrasive action of your scrub will be.

For normal skin, grind the pits to a loose powder similar to corn meal in texture. If the skin needs more abrasiveness, grind the pits to a consistency closer to oatmeal. For less abrasive action, powder the pits to a fine dust.

The product will have its own natural scent and color, but if you desire a specific fragrance color to suit your needs or an aromatherapy benefit you may add your favorite colorant or essential oils to the recipe.

While I do add herbs & oils that contain beneficial compounds, I typically do not add color or fragrance to any product designed for damaged skin because additives can cause the irritation to worsen.

You can use the scrubs alone or mix them with a cold cream or soap for a foaming action. You may also place your ground pits in a scrubbing bag for easier and cleaner application. Just be sure your chosen bag has large enough mesh to allow the pits abrasive action to come through.

Remember that everyone's skin reacts differently. You should test the products on a less sensitive area before using them.

Daily Scrub

This is a nice base exfoliation recipe. You can use this recipe as it is written or you can customize this base to suit almost any cleansing need. I try to use this cleanser once or twice a week to help reveal better-looking skin, allow penetration of the compounds of my other cleansing products and improve my skins overall texture.

1 tbsp. Scrubbing Agent of your choice

Almonds Powder (rougher skin)

Oatmeal or Cornmeal (gentle cleansing)

Ground Citrus Peels (clarifying)

1 tbsp. Rose Water

1 tsp. Honey

Emulsifier & Thickener as desired

Mix all of the ingredients in a blender until well blended but not slush.

Store the finished product in a clean container with a tight fitting lid. This mixture may separate so shake it well before each use.

While I do add herbs & oils that contain beneficial compounds, I typically do not add color or fragrance to any product designed for damaged skin because additives can cause the irritation to worsen. This recipe has a fresh clean smell and a light color. If you desire a different color or fragrance, you may add your favorite colorant or essential oils or herbs to the mixture.

Remember that everyone's skin reacts differently. You should test the products on a less sensitive area before using them.

Gentle Dermabrasion Scrub

This mildly abrasive cleanser helps to remove surface dirt, oils, and dead skin cells through a gentle cleansing action without the harsh effects of some other abrasives. This recipe includes my favorite ingredients but you might want to refer to the appendix for ingredient ideas that will work better with your personal acne needs.

1 cup Distilled Water

1 tsp. Elderberry

Bring the water to a light boil. Remove the water from the heat. Add the blackthorn flowers. Allow the mixture to steep for about 6 hours to create a strong infusion. Strain the elderberry from the mixture. The liquid will act as a base for your recipe. Add

1/2 cup Uncooked Oatmeal

1/2 tsp. Evening Primrose Oil

1 tbsp. Glycerin

2 drops Tincture of Benzoin

Emulsifier & Thickener as desired

Place all of the ingredients in a blender or food processor and mix for approximately 2 minutes until a pasty texture has been achieved.

While I do add herbs & oils that contain beneficial compounds, I typically do not add color or fragrance to any product designed for damaged skin because additives can cause the irritation to worsen. If you prefer something other than the natural color or scent, you can add your favorite colorant, essential oils or herbs to the mixture.

Store the finished product in a clean container with a tight fitting lid. This mixture may separate so shake it well before each use. Massage a small amount into skin with a gentle upward motion. Allow the mixture to sit on the skin for 60 seconds before rinsing well.

This gentle cleanser works well for all skin types. This mixture may be used on the face and body.

Experiment by adding specialized ingredients to suit your skin needs

For a foaming effect, you can add 2 tbsp. of coconut oil to the recipe.

Remember that everyone's skin reacts differently. You should test the products on a less sensitive area before using them.

Rough Skin Grain Bag

This grain mixture is one of my favorites for use in scrubbing sacks. The grains gently exfoliate and the oils infuse the newly bared skin with moisture. This blend works especially well on rougher areas like the elbows and the feet. These areas often need special attention and this recipe combines the treatment steps into one easy application.

1/4 tsp. Borax Powder

1 tsp. Ground Sage

1/4 cup Oatmeal

1/4 cup Cornmeal

1 tsp. Honey

1/4 cup Wheat Germ Oil

Place all of the dry ingredients in a blender or food processor. Mix for approximately 2 minutes until the ingredients are smooth.

Pour the oils and honey over the dry ingredients and mix again to distribute the oils evenly.

Place 3-4 tbsp. of the mixture on your favorite scrub sack.

The product will have its own natural scent and color, but if you desire a specific color to suit your needs or an aromatherapy benefit you may add your favorite colorant or essential oils to the recipe. While I do add herbs & oils that contain beneficial compounds, I typically do not add color or fragrance to any product designed for damaged skin because additives can cause the irritation to worsen. If you prefer something other than the natural color or scent, you can add your favorite colorant, essential oils or herbs to the mixture.

To use, moisten the scrub sack and use it as you would soap. I use this bag specifically on the rough, dry patches of my skin but it works well all over the body and face. Dry the bag between uses to ensure the longest shelf life possible.

Experiment by adding specialized ingredients to suit your skin needs.

For a foaming effect, you can add 2 tbsp. of coconut oil to the recipe.

Remember that everyone's skin reacts differently. You should test the products on a less sensitive area before using them.

Intense Skin Scrub

Some areas of the body might need a more intense exfoliation action. This scrub is a bit harsher and should not be used on the face or sensitive areas. I find this recipe to be useful for my feet & elbows especially during the winter months when dry skin build up can be more of a problem.

3 tbsp. Almond Oil

2 tbsp. Ground Almond (almond meal may be used if desired)

1/4 cup Aloe Vera Gel

3 tbsp. Witch Hazel Gel

Place the aloe & ground almond in a blender or food processor. Mix for approximately 2 minutes until the ingredients are smooth.

Pour the oils and witch hazel over the dry ingredients and mix the scrub again to ensure an even distribution of all of the ingredients.

Place 3-4 tbsp. of the mixture on your favorite scrub sack.

The product will have its own natural scent and color, but if you desire a specific color to suit your needs or an aromatherapy benefit you may add your favorite colorant or essential oils to the recipe. While I do add herbs & oils that contain beneficial compounds, I typically do not add color or fragrance to any product designed for damaged skin because additives can cause the irritation to worsen. If you prefer something other than the natural color or scent, you can add your favorite colorant, essential oils or herbs to the mixture.

To use, moisten the scrub sack and use it as you would soap. I use this bag specifically on the rough, dry patches of my skin but it works well all over the body and face. Dry the bag between uses to ensure the longest shelf life possible.

Experiment by adding specialized ingredients to suit your skin needs

For a foaming effect, you can add 2 tbsp. of coconut oil to the recipe.

If the mixture is courser than desired, you may place all of the ingredients in the blender and gently blend until the desired consistency is reached.

Remember that everyone's skin reacts differently. You should test the products on a less sensitive area before using them.

Toning Scrub

This mildly abrasive scrub works well as a toning agent and is a great option to help exfoliate her skin while achieving a younger, more toned look and feel.

1/2 Finely Chopped Cucumber (including peel)

2 tbsp. Jojoba Oil

2 tbsp. Cucumber Juice

1 tsp. Lemon Juice

1/8 cup Rose Water

1/8 cup Witch Hazel

Emulsifier & Thickener as desired

Mix all of the ingredients in a blender until they are well blended but not slush.

While I do add herbs & oils that contain beneficial compounds, I typically do not add color or fragrance to any product designed for damaged skin because additives can cause the irritation to worsen. If you prefer something other than the natural color or scent, you can add your favorite colorant, essential oils, or herbs to the mixture.

Store the finished product in a clean container with a tight fitting lid. This mixture may separate so shake it well before each use.

Remember that everyone's skin reacts differently. You should test the products on a less sensitive area before using them.

Daily Wrinkle Reduction Scrub

This gentle cleanser helps to add moisture to the skin while reducing the appearance of fine lines & wrinkles. It is gentle enough for daily use.

1/4 cup Cornstarch

2 tbsp. Witch Hazel

2 tbsp Grapeseed Oil

1 tsp. Evening Primrose Oil

1 tsp. Spikenard

Emulsifier & Thickener as desired

Place all of the ingredients in the blender or food processor and whip the mixture until the ingredients are well blended.

While I do add herbs & oils that contain beneficial compounds, I typically do not add color or fragrance to any product designed for damaged skin because additives can cause the irritation to worsen. If you prefer something other than the natural color or scent, you can add your favorite colorant, essential oils, or herbs to the mixture.

Spoon the cleanser into a clean container and seal it tightly.

To use, scoop a small amount into your hands and massage into your skin with gentle upward motions. Allow the scrub to sit on the skin for 60 seconds before rinsing.

Remember that everyone's skin reacts differently. You should test the products on a less sensitive area before using them.

Mermaid Bath Rub

Mermaids are said to have beautiful, glowing skin. Maybe this is because of the salt water that they call home. This treatment is very popular in the spas of the United States and Europe. The rub gently removes surface dirt and dead skin cells and then leaves the newly revealed skin in a condition where it can easily absorb the beneficial compounds of post-bath treatments. This treatment can cause additional irritation to damaged skin so only use this if your skin is already in good condition or if you have completed a test to make certain you will not have a bad reaction to the scrub.

1/2 cup Sea Salt

1/2 cup Epsom Salts

1/2 cup Apricot Kernel Oil

1 tsp. Vitamin E Oil

Mix the salts and oils until they are well blended. They will form a thick paste.

The product will have its own natural scent and color, but if you desire a specific color to suit your needs or an aromatherapy benefit you may add your favorite colorant, essential oils or herbs to the recipe.

While I do add herbs & oils that contain beneficial compounds, I typically do not add color or fragrance to any product designed for damaged skin because additives can cause the irritation to worsen.

Spoon the paste into a clean container and seal it tightly.

To use, massage a handful of the paste into your skin starting at the top of your body and working your way toward your feet. This treatment is not recommended for use on the face or neck.

When you reach your feet, rinse your skin well and pat it dry.

Do not use soap following this treatment because it will minimize the effects.

Be very careful because the oils will make your skin and tub very slippery.

Remember that everyone's skin reacts differently. You should test the products on a less sensitive area before using them.

Citrus Scrub

This scrub has a clean scent and provides moisture to dry, rough skin while gently removing dead cells. I like to use this in combination with some of my other citrus-based products to provide an all over body theme to the day. The oils are rich in oils and anti-oxidants while the juices provide a wonderful clarifying action.

1 tsp. Lemon Juice

1/4 tso. Borax Powder

1/4 cup Pineapple Juice

1/4 cup Jojoba Oil

1/4 cup Aloe Vera Gel

1 Orange or Lemon Peel – finely ground

Blend the ingredients until they are well mixed.

The product will have its own natural scent and color, but if you desire a specific color to suit your needs or an aromatherapy benefit you may add your favorite colorant, oils or herbs to the recipe.

While I do add herbs & oils that contain beneficial compounds, I typically do not add color or fragrance to any product designed for damaged skin because additives can cause the irritation to worsen. If you prefer something other than the natural color or scent, you can add your favorite colorant, essential oils, or herbs to the mixture.

Pour the scrub into a clean container and seal it tightly. Store the unused scrub in the refrigerator to extend its shelf life.

To apply, shake the mixture well and massage a handful into your skin.

I like to follow this treatment with a citrus scented lotion for extra conditioning.

Remember that everyone's skin reacts differently. You should test the products on a less sensitive area before using them.

Brightening Scrub

This brightening scrub helps to add luster to the skin and restore the radiant glow that adds beauty to skin of any age.

1 Whole Strawberry

1/4 cup Cucumber Juice

1 tsp. Angelica

1 tsp. Geranium Oil

2 tsp. Witch Hazel

Emulsifier & Thickener as desired

Whip all of the ingredients in a blender or by hand until they are well blended.

This is a very loose and liquid cleanser and may be more difficult to apply. You can select a beneficial thickening agent like Arrowroot or Acacia Powder to add to the recipe if you prefer.

This mixture will have a reddish color and a clean scent. While I do add herbs & oils that contain beneficial compounds, I typically do not add color or fragrance to any product designed for damaged skin because additives can cause the irritation to worsen. If you prefer something other than the natural color or scent, you can add your favorite colorant, essential oils, or herbs to the mixture.

Pour a small amount in the palm of your hand, massage gently into the skin using an upward motion. This cleanser should be allowed to set into the skin for at least 1 minute before rinsing.

Store the extra cleanser in the refrigerator between uses.

Remember that everyone's skin reacts differently. You should test the products on a less sensitive area before using them.

Astringents & Toners

Astringents & Toners are an essential element to maintaining healthy skin. They work with your cleansers and scrubs to help to keep the skin free of dirt and oils. Astringents & toners are a fantastic choice to help to get rid of the residue that cleansers sometimes leave behind.

Astringents and toners also help to minimize the appearance of pores. You should select astringent and toner recipes that complement your other daily care regimen components. I like to choose a toner to use throughout the day to keep my skin looking and feeling fresh.

Remember that everyone's skin reacts differently. You should test the products on a less sensitive area before using them.

Basic Astringent

This is a great basic astringent for every day needs. It works very well as the recipe is written but it also makes an excellent base for custom astringent products designed to suit your specific needs.

5 tbsp Rosewater

You may substitute distilled water if preferred

1 tbsp Witch Hazel

1/8 tsp. Borax Powder

Dissolve the borax power in the rose water. You may need to heat the rose water slightly to help dissolve the borax powder. Do not boil the rose water since this can cause some of the beneficial compound to be destroyed and will result in some evaporation.

Add the witch hazel and stir the mixture until it is well blended.

You may want to select additives and ingredients from your natural care kit to strengthen or alter the affect of the toner. You should decide what ingredients best suit your skin care goals and add them accordingly. You do not have to add any other compounds if you do not need enhanced treatments since this toner works very well alone.

While I do add herbs & oils that contain beneficial compounds, I typically do not add color or fragrance to any product designed for damaged skin because additives can cause the irritation to worsen. If you prefer something other than the natural color or scent, you can add your favorite colorant, essential oils, or herbs to the mixture.

Store the finished toner in an airtight container to prevent evaporation. Apply the toner to your skin using a clean cotton ball. Do not rinse this recipe from your skin. Allow the liquid to dry naturally and continue to work throughout the day. You can use moisturizer & makeup after the liquid has dried.

Remember that everyone's skin reacts differently. You should test the products on a less sensitive area before using them.

Juicy Juice Astringent

Juices from apples, cherries, plums or berries contain natural humectants that attract moisture and provide a smooth texture to the skin. This is one of my favorite astringent products because it helps to keep my skin fresh while promoting a healthy, moisturized appearance.

1/2 cup Juice of Choice

3 tbsp. Rosewater

3 tbsp. Witch Hazel

Blend all of the ingredients.

Pour the ingredients directly into the airtight storage container. Shake the mixture well to blend all of the ingredients.

While I do add herbs & oils that contain beneficial compounds, I typically do not add color or fragrance to any product designed for damaged skin because additives can cause the irritation to worsen. If you prefer something other than the natural color or scent, you can add your favorite colorant, essential oils, or herbs to the mixture.

This recipe may separate so shake it well before each use. You may wish to store this recipe in the refrigerator to extend the shelf life. Do not rinse this recipe from your skin. Allow the liquid to dry naturally and continue to work throughout the day. You can use moisturizer & makeup after the liquid has dried.

Remember that everyone's skin reacts differently. You should test the products on a less sensitive area before using them.

Smoothing & Toning Astringent

This is an excellent toner to help smooth & tone overstressed skin. It works equally well on the face and body.

1 cup Distilled Water

1/2 tsp. Spikenard

1/2 tsp. Basil Leaves

1/2 cup Witch Hazel

Bring the water to a light boil and remove it from the heat. Add the flowers and leaves to the hot water. Steep the flowers & leaves in the water for up to 24 hours or until you achieve a nice dark brew. Strain the flowers and leaves from the fluid and discard the plant parts. The fluid will act as the base for your toner.

Stir witch hazel into the liquid base.

While I do add herbs & oils that contain beneficial compounds, I typically do not add color or fragrance to any product designed for damaged skin because additives can cause the irritation to worsen. If you prefer something other than the natural color or scent, you can add your favorite colorant, essential oils, or herbs to the mixture.

Pour the finished toner into your favorite spray or dispenser bottle. Seal the container tightly to prevent evaporation.

Apply the finished product to your skin using a cotton ball or spritzer

Do not rinse this recipe from your skin. Allow the liquid to dry naturally and continue to work throughout the day. You can use moisturizer & makeup after the liquid has dried.

Remember that everyone's skin reacts differently. You should test the products on a less sensitive area before using them.

Brightening Toner

This toner helps to wake up dull skin, speed healing, and reduce the dullness that can contribute to an aged look. It works equally well on the face and body.

1 cup Distilled Water

1/2 tsp. Carob Powder

1/2 tsp. Basil Leaves

1/2 cup Orange Flower Water

Bring the water to a light boil and remove it from the heat. Add the powder and leaves to the hot water. Steep the flowers & leaves in the water for up to 24 hours or until you achieve a nice dark brew. Strain the leaves from the fluid and discard the plant parts. The fluid will act as the base for your toner.

Stir the orange flower water into the liquid base.

While I do add herbs & oils that contain beneficial compounds, I typically do not add color or fragrance to any product designed for damaged skin because additives can cause the irritation to worsen. If you prefer something other than the natural color or scent, you can add your favorite colorant, essential oils, or herbs to the mixture.

Pour the finished toner into your favorite spray or dispenser bottle. Seal the container tightly to prevent evaporation.

Apply the finished product to your skin using a cotton ball or spritzer.

Do not rinse this recipe from your skin. Allow the liquid to dry naturally and continue to work throughout the day. You can use moisturizer & makeup after the liquid has dried.

Remember that everyone's skin reacts differently. You should test the products on a less sensitive area before using them.

Alternative Brightening Toner

Dull & dark skin can be one of the hardest things to combat. This wonderful brightening toner works well in combination with a brightening cleanser & lotion combination to wake up dingy skin and leave your skin looking great.

1/4 cup Distilled Water

1 tbsp. Chamomile

4 tbsp. Rosewater

1 tbsp. Lemon

Bring the water to a light boil and remove it from the heat. Add the chamomile to the hot water. Steep the chamomile in the water for up to 24 hours or until you achieve a nice dark brew. Strain the leaves from the fluid and discard the plant parts. The fluid will act as the base for your toner.

Stir witch hazel into the liquid base.

While I do add herbs & oils that contain beneficial compounds, I typically do not add color or fragrance to any product designed for damaged skin because additives can cause the irritation to worsen. If you prefer something other than the natural color or scent, you can add your favorite colorant, essential oils, or herbs to the mixture.

Pour the finished toner into your favorite spray or dispenser bottle. Seal the container tightly to prevent evaporation.

Apply the finished product to your skin using a cotton ball or spritzer.

Do not rinse this recipe from your skin. Allow the liquid to dry naturally and continue to work throughout the day. You can use moisturizer & makeup after the liquid has dried.

Remember that everyone's skin reacts differently. You should test the products on a less sensitive area before using them.

Healing Toner

Honey is one of my favorite skin care ingredients. It not only helps to soften the skin, it also has antibacterial and healing properties. This toner works well for anyone who has skin irritation since it softens, heals, and tones all in one-step.

2 tbsp. Honey

4 tbsp. Strong Chamomile Tea

4 tbsp. Rosewater

2 tbsp. Honey

4 tbsp. Strong Chamomile Tea

4 tbsp. Rose Water

You can make the chamomile tea using 1 tbsp. of chamomile and ½ cup water. Bring the water to a boil and then remove it from the heat. Add the chamomile. Allow the mixture to steep up to 24 hours or until a strong tea has been created. Strain the plant parts from the fluid.

Blend all of the ingredients directly into the container you will use as a dispenser.

While I do add herbs & oils that contain beneficial compounds, I typically do not add color or fragrance to any product designed for damaged skin because additives can cause the irritation to worsen. If you prefer something other than the natural color or scent, you can add your favorite colorant, essential oils, or herbs to the mixture.

The toner will be sticky at first. Aging helps to diminish the sticky quality. I like to age this toner for about 1 week before use but you can use it immediately if you wish.

Do not rinse this recipe from your skin. Allow the liquid to dry naturally and continue to work throughout the day. You can use moisturizer & makeup after the liquid has dried.

Remember that everyone's skin reacts differently. You should test the products on a less sensitive area before using them.

Cooling Toner

Cucumber juice is known for its ability to relieve sore skin, sooth inflammation and speed healing while reducing puffiness. This toner has one of the cleanest scents and is a favorite of everyone in the house.

1/2 cup Cucumber Juice

4 tbsp. Witch Hazel

2 tbsp. Rose Water

You can make cucumber juice by chopping the cucumber, including the peel into smaller pieces. Place the pieces into the blender and whip on a medium setting until the pieces are pulped. Strain off the green juice for use in the recipe.

Add the remaining ingredients to the cucumber juice and mix until they are well blended.

While I do add herbs & oils that contain beneficial compounds, I typically do not add color or fragrance to any product designed for damaged skin because additives can cause the irritation to worsen. If you prefer something other than the natural color or scent, you can add your favorite colorant, essential oils, or herbs to the mixture.

Store the completed toner in an airtight container. You may wish to place the container in the refrigerator to increase the shelf life of the finished product.

Do not rinse this recipe from your skin. Allow the liquid to dry naturally and continue to work throughout the day. You can use moisturizer & makeup after the liquid has dried.

Remember that everyone's skin reacts differently. You should test the products on a less sensitive area before using them.

Restorative Toner

This nice restorative toner helps to speed healing, combat bacteria, and promote clear skin. It is a nice toning choice for those whose skin is fatigued and for use by acne sufferers whose skin is beginning to age.

1 tsp. Honey

1 tsp. Evening Primrose Oil

1 tsp. Finely Ground Immortelle

3 tbsp. Aloe Vera Gel

1/4 cup Witch Hazel

Whip the ingredients until they are well blended.

While I do add herbs & oils that contain beneficial compounds, I typically do not add color or fragrance to any product designed for damaged skin because additives can cause the irritation to worsen. If you prefer something other than the natural color or scent, you can add your favorite colorant, essential oils, or herbs to the mixture.

Store the completed toner in an airtight container.

The toner will be sticky at first. Aging helps to diminish the sticky quality. I like to age this toner about 1 week before use but you can use it immediately if you wish.

Do not rinse this recipe from your skin. Allow the liquid to dry naturally and continue to work throughout the day. You can use moisturizer & makeup after the liquid has dried.

Remember that everyone's skin reacts differently. You should test the products on a less sensitive area before using them.

Gentle Astringent for Sensitive Skin

Aging sometimes increases skin sensitivity making the products that we choose to use for skin cleansing especially important. Many of the more common treatments are harsh and can damage sensitive skin. This nice toner helps to promote clear, fresh looking skin without creating irritation.

4 tbsp. Rosewater

4 tbsp. Orange Flower Water

2 tbsp. Aloe Vera

Pour the liquids directly into a spray bottle. Shake the bottle well to blend the ingredients.

While I do add herbs & oils that contain beneficial compounds, I typically do not add color or fragrance to any product designed for damaged skin because additives can cause the irritation to worsen. If you prefer something other than the natural color or scent, you can add your favorite colorant, essential oils, or herbs to the mixture.

Shake the completed toner well before each use. Do not rinse this recipe from your skin. Allow the liquid to dry naturally and continue to work throughout the day. You can use moisturizer & makeup after the liquid has dried.

Remember that everyone's skin reacts differently. You should test the products on a less sensitive area before using them.

Scar Reduction Toner

Aging, acne, and exposure to the sun can create dark pigmentation spots on the skin. This is a nice toner to use on a regular basis to help reduce the appearance of light pitting and hyper-pigmentation while keeping the skin free of dirt, oils, and toxins.

4 tbsp. Rosewater

4 tbsp. Powdered Avens

4 tbsp. Papaya Milk

Pour the ingredients directly into a spray bottle. Add the powdered Avens and shake the bottle until the ingredients are well blended. You may need to heat the ingredients a bit to help the powder dissolve.

While I do add herbs & oils that contain beneficial compounds, I typically do not add color or fragrance to any product designed for damaged skin because additives can cause the irritation to worsen. If you prefer something other than the natural color or scent, you can add your favorite colorant, essential oils, or herbs to the mixture.

Shake the completed toner well before each use. Do not rinse this recipe from your skin. Allow the liquid to dry naturally and continue to work throughout the day. You can use moisturizer & makeup after the liquid has dried.

Remember that everyone's skin reacts differently. You should test the products on a less sensitive area before using them.

Deep Bath Treatments & Masks

Sometimes a deep treatment helps to maximize the benefits of daily care. At other times, deep treatments are necessary to start the healing processes and remove obstacles that can interfere with your selected daily cleansing & moisturizing plans.

Deep treatments are designed to deliver concentrated benefits to a specific area helping to achieve results much more quickly. Deep treatments should not be overused since they tend to be more concentrated and overuse can actually cause more damage than benefit.

Masks & deep treatments help to pamper your skin and prepare it for a daily regimen that will aid you in achieving healthy, younger looking skin.

While I do add herbs & oils that contain beneficial compounds, I typically do not add color or fragrance to any product designed for damaged skin because additives can cause the irritation to worsen. If you prefer something other than the natural color or scent, you can add your favorite colorant, essential oils, or herbs to the recipes.

Remember that everyone's skin reacts differently. You should test the products on a less sensitive area before using them.

Steam Treatment

One of the most effective daily treatments for clear, healthy looking skin is a steam treatment.

There are many machines available for steam treatments but they are not necessary for using steam & herbs to help open your pores and clean your skin.

You can use a stainless steel or other pot that does not have a coating that will release chemicals into the liquid as it boils.

2 cups Distilled Water

1 tsp. Bay Leaves

1 tsp. Spearmint Leaves

You can add the herbs loose or use a tea ball to contain the plant parts.

Place a clean, cotton towel over the top of the pan.

Bring the water & herb mixture to a light boil.

Gently lift the edge of the towel to direct the steam.

Use your hand to test the temperature of the steam before putting your face into the flow. Your hand will help you to find the distance that gives you warm but not hot steam.

Place your face in the stream of steam.

Relax and allow the moisture and plant compounds to do their job.

When you are finished, rinse your face with cool water and gently pat it dry.

Collagen Building Mask

Gelatin is one of my favorite mask bases for aging skin. It is not as drawing as clay and it helps to attract moisture while the other ingredients cleanse and fight the signs of aging. This treatment helps to build collagen, infuse moisture, and reduce fine lines.

1/2 cup Gelatin – 1 packet

1/2 cup Distilled Water

1/2 tsp. Myrrh

1/2 tsp. Borage Seed Oil

Mix the gelatin and water until they are well blended.

Before the gelatin hardens, stir in the remaining ingredients.

The product will have its own natural scent and color, but if you desire a specific color to suit your needs or an aromatherapy benefit you may add your favorite colorant or essential oils to the recipe. While I do add herbs & oils that contain beneficial compounds, I typically do not add color or fragrance to any product designed for damaged skin because additives can cause the irritation to worsen.

To use, apply the mixture to your skin in an even coat.

Allow the mixture to soak into your skin for approximately 30 minutes or until the gelatin is completely dry.

Peel or rinse the mask from your skin.

Remember that everyone's skin reacts differently. You should test the products on a less sensitive area before using them.

Toning Wrap

This wrap helps to reduce the appearance of pores while toning the skin. I love to use a wrap like this as often as I can in the summer because summer wear can show off every flaw or it can show off beautiful toned skin!

1/4 cup Elderberry Juice

1/4 cup Distilled Water

1/4 tsp. Cypress Oil

1/2 cup Kaolin Clay

1 tbsp. Carob Powder

Mix the juice and the water. Dissolve the carob powders in the liquid solution. Add the oils to the mixture stirring until it is distributed evenly.

Slowly add the clay powder until a thick paste is formed. You do not want the mixture to be too wet since it may be difficult to apply. If it is too firm, add a few extra dashes of clay until it reaches the desired consistency. If it is too firm, you can add a few drops of water until you get the consistency you want.

The product will have its own natural scent and color, but if you desire a specific color to suit your needs or an aromatherapy benefit you may add your favorite colorant or essential oils to the recipe. While I do add herbs & oils that contain beneficial compounds, I typically do not add color or fragrance to any product designed for damaged skin because additives can cause the irritation to worsen.

To use, apply the mixture to your skin in an even coat.

Allow the mixture to soak into your skin for approximately 30 minutes or until the gelatin is completely dry.

Rinse the wrap from your skin and follow it with a healing moisturizing treatment.

Remember that everyone's skin reacts differently. You should test the products on a less sensitive area before using them.

Aloe Vera Healing Wrap

Aloe Vera is a wonderful treatment for many, many problems. Perhaps one of the best uses is to sooth skin irritation while supporting collagen-building mechanisms. Palmarosa and Galbanum are two of my favorite additives but you can select almost any other powder or oil from the appendix list to include in your personal healing wrap.

1/4 cup Powdered Clay – Kaolin works best

1/4 cup Aloe Vera Gel

1 tbsp. Palmarosa Oil

1 tbsp. Galbanum Oil

Blend the oils and slowly add them to the aloe vera base, stirring well to ensure that you have an even distribution.

Slowly stir in the clay until the mixture forms a thick paste. If the mixture is too dry, you can add a few drops of orange flower water until the desired consistency is obtained.

The product will have its own natural scent and color, but if you desire a specific color to suit your needs or an aromatherapy benefit you may add your favorite colorant or essential oils to the recipe. While I do add herbs & oils that contain beneficial compounds, I typically do not add color or fragrance to any product designed for damaged skin because additives can cause the irritation to worsen.

To use, apply the mixture to your skin in an even coat.

Allow the mixture to soak into your skin for approximately 30 minutes or until the clay is completely dry.

Rinse the wrap from your skin and follow it with a healing moisturizing treatment.

Remember that everyone's skin reacts differently. You should test the products on a less sensitive area before using them.

Gelatin Brightening Mask

Gelatin works wonders for attracting moisture and helping the additives in a mask recipe to infuse their benefits into the skin. This mask is wonderful for hydrating and brightening dull skin while giving it the nourishment it needs to look & feel its best.

1/2 cup Gelatin – 1 packet

1/2 cup Distilled Water

1/2 tsp. Lemon Juice

1/2 tsp. Angelica Oil

Mix the gelatin and water until they are well blended.

Before the gelatin hardens, stir in the remaining ingredients.

If the mixture is too thick, you can add a few drops of warm water until the mixture reaches your preferred consistency. If the mixture is too loose, allow the gelatin to solidify a bit longer before using the mask.

The product will have its own natural scent and color, but if you desire a specific color to suit your needs or an aromatherapy benefit you may add your favorite colorant or essential oils to the recipe. While I do add herbs & oils that contain beneficial compounds, I typically do not add color or fragrance to any product designed for damaged skin because additives can cause the irritation to worsen.

To use, apply the mixture to your skin in an even coat.

Allow the mixture to soak into your skin for approximately 30 minutes or until the gelatin is completely dry.

Peel or rinse the mask from your skin.

Remember that everyone's skin reacts differently. You should test the products on a less sensitive area before using them.

Seborrhea Soothing Mask

No matter what age we are, acne and seborrhea can be a problem. This is a fantastic mask to reduce the appearance of outbreaks while acting to prevent future issues. Henna comes in colored and colorless forms and you will want to be sure that you are using colorless henna powder unless you are hoping to make a sunless tanning product out of your wrap!

1/2 cup Colorless Henna Powder

1/4 cup Witch Hazel

1/4 cup Distilled Water

2 tbsp. Powdered Lemongrass

Stir the lemongrass and henna powders until they are well blended.

Slowly add the blended powders to the liquid until the ingredients form a thick paste. If the mixture is too liquid, you can add a bit more henna powder. If the mixture it too solid, you can add a few extra drops of witch hazel.

The product will have its own natural scent and color, but if you desire a specific color to suit your needs or an aromatherapy benefit you may add your favorite colorant or essential oils to the recipe. While I do add herbs & oils that contain beneficial compounds, I typically do not add color or fragrance to any product designed for damaged skin because additives can cause the irritation to worsen.

To use, apply the mixture to your skin in an even coat.

Allow the mixture to soak into your skin for approximately 30 minutes or until the gelatin is completely dry.

Rinse the mask from your skin and follow with a hydrating moisturizer.

Remember that everyone's skin reacts differently. You should test the products on a less sensitive area before using them.

Skin Renewal Body Mask

This body-mask is very popular in day spas. The mask extracts toxins from below the surface of the skin and leaves a beautiful clear glow behind. I love to use this recipe at least once a month to keep my skin clear and glowing.

1/4 cup Distilled Water

3 tbsp. Jojoba Oil

1/4 cup Aloe Vera Gel

Whip the water, aloe vera gel, and oil until they are well blended. Add

1/4 cup Powdered Kelp (seaweed)

2 tbsp. Sea Salt

Stir the mixture until the salts and powders are evenly distributed in the base.

1/2 cup Powdered Clay

Slowly add the clay powder until the mixture forms a thick paste.

If the powder is too dry and flaky, add a few extra drops of distilled water until the mask reaches the desired texture. If the mask is too moist, add a few extra dashes of clay until the mixture firms enough for easy application.

The product will have its own natural scent and color, but if you desire a specific color to suit your needs or an aromatherapy benefit you may add your favorite colorant or essential oils to the recipe. While I do add herbs & oils that contain beneficial compounds, I typically do not add color or fragrance to any product designed for damaged skin because additives can cause the irritation to worsen.

To use, apply the paste to your skin in an even coat.

Allow the mixture to soak into your skin for approximately 30 minutes or until it is completely dry.

Peel the mixture from the skin, rinse well, and pat the skin dry.

Remember that everyone's skin reacts differently. You should test the products on a less sensitive area before using them.

Fountain of Youth Bath

This wonderful bath additive is fantastic for people of all ages. The chamomile and carrot juice aid in hydrating while the oils gently bath your skin in moisture. The combination of seaweed and alum powder helps tighten and tone her skin giving it a hydrated and youthful glow.

1 tsp. Dried Chamomile (1 teabag)

1/2 cup Boiling Water

Bring the water to a light boil and remove it from the heat. Pour the water over the chamomile leaves and allow the mixture to soak overnight. You should have a strong tea. Strain the leaves from the liquid and discard them. The liquid will act as your recipe base.

1/4 cup Carrot

1/8 cup Seaweed Powder

1/2 cup Wheat Germ Oil

1 tsp. Alum Powder

Use only *USP Grade for Cosmetic Use* Alum Powder. Do not use metal when working with Alum Powder.

Blend all of the ingredients.

Pour the finished mixture into a clean container and seal it tightly.

The product will have its own natural scent and color, but if you desire a specific color to suit your needs or an aromatherapy benefit you may add your favorite colorant or essential oils to the recipe. While I do add herbs & oils that contain beneficial compounds, I typically do not add color or fragrance to any product designed for damaged skin because additives can cause the irritation to worsen.

Shake the mixture well before each use.

To use, add approximately 1/8 cup to warm bathwater and soak for 10-15 minutes.

Remember that everyone's skin reacts differently. You should test the products on a less sensitive area before using them.

Hydrating Soak

This wonderfully hydrating bath soak helps to increase collagen production, reduce skin inflammation, and combat the most common causes of environmental aging.

1/4 cup Aloe Vera Gel

1 tbsp. Vitamin E Oil

2 tbsp. Powdered Milk

1/4 cup Apricot Kernel Oil

Blend all of the ingredients in a clean container with a tight fitting lid.

The product will have its own natural scent and color, but if you desire a specific color to suit your needs or an aromatherapy benefit you may add your favorite colorant or essential oils to the recipe. While I do add herbs & oils that contain beneficial compounds, I typically do not add color or fragrance to any product designed for damaged skin because additives can cause the irritation to worsen.

Shake the mixture well before each use since the ingredients may separate if allowed to sit.

To use, add approximately 1/8 cup to warm bathwater and soak for 10-15 minutes.

Remember that everyone's skin reacts differently. You should test the products on a less sensitive area before using them.

Simple Hydrating Bath

When working to combat the signs of aging, it is easy to forget that well-hydrated skin is critical to the success of any other treatments. Well-hydrated skin will be better able to absorb the daily treatments, resist aging more effectively, and look healthier.

1 tbsp. Chamomile Leaves

1 tbsp. Basil Leaves

1 cup Boiling Distilled Water

Bring the water to a light boil and remove it from the heat. Pour the boiling water over the leaves and allow the mixture to steep overnight.

Strain the leaves from the fluid. Add

1/4 cup Carrot Juice

1/4 cup Tomato Juice (without seeds)

Stir the mixture until the ingredients are well blended.

Your recipe will be an orange tone and have a slight aroma. If you wish, you can use colorants, herbs, or oils to alter the color or fragrance.

While I do add herbs & oils that contain beneficial compounds, I typically do not add color or fragrance to any product designed for damaged skin because additives can cause the irritation to worsen. If you prefer something other than the natural color or scent, you can add your favorite colorant, essential oils, or herbs to the mixture.

Pour the finished mixture into your favorite tightly sealed container.

To use, pour ½ of the mixture into a warm bath and soak 15-20 minutes.

Remember that everyone's skin reacts differently. You should test the products on a less sensitive area before using them.

Skin Clarifying Soak

Sometimes the root of dull looking skin is a concentration of built up dead skin and oils. Using a deep-treatment clarifying product once a month helps to reduce the amount of surface dirt, oils, & toxins that remain after your daily regimen. This soak is one of my favorites because it leaves the skin hydrated & healthy while giving me the full body treatment I need to help my daily care regimen work at its best.

1/4 cup Vinegar

1 cup Orange Flower Water

1/2 cup Rose Water

1/4 cup Sea Salts

Dissolve the salts in the liquid base and shake solution until well blended.

The recipe will have a stronger vinegar smell so you may want to add your favorite fragrances to your solution to alter the smell.

Food coloring may also be added to provide a pretty color to your recipe and your bath Water. The vinegar smell will fade from your skin very quickly so scent is not necessary to the recipe.

While do add herbs & oils that contain beneficial compounds, I typically do not add color or fragrance to any product designed for damaged skin because additives can cause the irritation to worsen. If you prefer something other than the natural color or scent, you can add your favorite colorant, essential oils, or herbs to the mixture.

Pour the finished product into a clean container and seal tightly.

You will want to shake the solution before using to ensure the ingredients are well blended.

To use add approximately ¼ cup of the mixture to your bath and soak approximately 15-20 minutes.

If your skin is not oily, you should follow this treatment with a light moisturizer.

Remember that everyone's skin reacts differently. You should test the products on a less sensitive area before using them.

Age Defying Bath Balm

This wonderful mixture is a favorite whenever I know I will be showing off my skin. It helps tighten & tone while preparing the skin for the moisturizer of choice. This particular recipe can irritate some people since it is contains ingredients that have a more extreme affect so make sure that you conduct a sensitivity test before using it.

2 cups Sea Salt

1 tbsp. Powdered Seaweed

4 tbsp. Powdered Clary Sage

Mix the dry ingredients until they are well blended. Add

1/4 cup Rosewater

2 tbsp. Sunflower Oil

1/8 cup Wheat Germ Oil

Combine the remaining ingredients with the liquid stirring until it is well blended.

While I do add herbs & oils that contain beneficial compounds, I typically do not add color or fragrance to any product designed for damaged skin because additives can cause the irritation to worsen. If you prefer something other than the natural color or scent, you can add your favorite colorant, essential oils, or herbs to the mixture.

Pour the finished mixture into a container and seal it tightly.

To use the bath, add 1/8 cup of the powdered solution to your warm bath water and soak until relief is obtained or 20-30 minutes.

Follow the treatment with a hydrating moisturizer for the best effect.

Remember that everyone's skin reacts differently. You should test the products on a less sensitive area before using them. You should also remember that even natural products have side effects.

Soothing Soak

This is an excellent choice for use when life is a bit stressful or the skin is irritated and sensitive. This soak helps to relax your mind and body while giving the skin a lustrous, silky feeling.

1/4 cup Aloe Vera Gel

1/4 cup Epsom Salts

4 tbsp. Lavender Oil

1/4 cup Apple Juice

1/4 cup Witch Hazel

Dissolve the salts in the witch hazel base.

Add the remaining ingredients and stir until they are well blended.

Pour the finished mixture into a clean container and seal it tightly.

Part of the benefit of this treatment comes from the scent released from the lavender oils. Some acne outbreaks are believed to be caused by stress. Lavender is both anti-bacterial and nervine making it a choice ingredient for treating acne. If you desire the skin benefits without the sedative and relaxing qualities of the lavender aroma, you may exchange the lavender with your favorite scent.

Food coloring may also be added at this time to create a pretty color to your recipe and the bath water.

While I do add herbs & oils that contain beneficial compounds, I typically do not add color or fragrance to any product designed for damaged skin because additives can cause the irritation to worsen.

This mixture may separate if left standing so you should shake the mixture well before each use.

To use, add approximately ¼ cup to warm bath water and soak for 10-15 minutes or until the desired soothing effect has been achieved.

Remember that everyone's skin reacts differently. You should test the products on a less sensitive area before using them.

Bath for Damaged Skin

This is an excellent balm for irritated or injured skin. I keep this mixed and available for use whenever my skin needs some extra special care. We have found this soak provides an excellent soothing bath if you have sunburn, eczema, or a rash.

1 tsp. Dried Marigold

1 tsp. Basil

1/2 cup Distilled Water

Bring the water to a boil and remove it from the heat. Pour the water over the marigold & basil. Allow the solution to steep 24 hours. Strain the plant parts from the water and discard the leaves. The fluid will be the base for the recipe.

2 tbsp. Almond Oil

2 tbsp. Coconut Oil

1 tbsp. Glycerin

2 tbsp. Honey Powder

3 tbsp. Aloe Vera Gel

Combine the remaining ingredients with the tea, stirring until they are well blended.

The mixture will have a wonderful aroma from the ingredients. While I do add herbs & oils that contain beneficial compounds, I typically do not add color or fragrance to any product designed for damaged skin because additives can cause the irritation to worsen. If you prefer something other than the natural color or scent, you can add your favorite colorant, essential oils, or herbs to the mixture.

Pour the finished mixture into a container and seal it tightly.

To use the bath, add ¼ cup of the liquid to your warm bath Water and soak until relief is obtained or 20-30 minutes.

You may need to repeat the process if the skin is especially irritated or sore.

For the best affect, follow the treatment with a soothing & healing moisturizer.

Remember that everyone's skin reacts differently. You should test the products on a less sensitive area before using them.

Youthful Milk Bath

Milk has long been believed to provide exceptional beauty benefits. This recipe combines the best of the milk and yogurt products with oils and humectants giving your skin the support it needs to stay healthy while providing a lovely moist glow. I use this bath as often as I can to give my skin a beautiful smooth texture.

1/4 cup Plain Yogurt

1/4 cup Powdered Milk

1 tbsp Wheat Germ Oil

1 tbsp. Glycerin

1 tbsp. Honey

Combine the ingredients in a clean container, stirring until they are well blended.

The mixture will have a wonderful aroma from the ingredients. While I do add herbs & oils that contain beneficial compounds, I typically do not add color or fragrance to any product designed for damaged skin because additives can cause the irritation to worsen. If you prefer something other than the natural color or scent, you can add your favorite colorant, essential oils, or herbs to the mixture.

Pour the finished mixture into a container and seal it tightly.

You will want to shake the solution before using to ensure the ingredients are well blended.

To use add approximately ¼ cup of the mixture to your bath and soak approximately 15-20 minutes.

Remember that everyone's skin reacts differently. You should test the products on a less sensitive area before using them.

Ivy Bath Soak

English Ivy is an excellent product for use when getting your skin ready for special occasions. The ivy helps draw fluids from the skin and reduces the appearance of acne, water retention, and other unsightly conditions. This mixture will tighten and tone the skin leaving it looking and feeling wonderful. You should not use this recipe for facial products.

10 English Ivy Leaves

1/2 cup Distilled Water

Heat the water to a light boil and remove it from the heat. Pour the heated water over the ivy leaves and allow the mixture to soak for 24 hours. Strain the leaves from the water and discard them. The fluid will act as the base for your recipe.

1/4 cup Jojoba Oil

3 tbsp Seaweed Powder

Add the oil and powder to your ivy Water and blend ingredients until they are well mixed.

While I do add herbs & oils that contain beneficial compounds, I typically do not add color or fragrance to any product designed for damaged skin because additives can cause the irritation to worsen. If you prefer something other than the natural color or scent, you can add your favorite colorant, essential oils, or herbs to the mixture.

Pour the completed solution into a clean container and seal it tightly.

To use, shake the mixture well and pour ¼ cup into your bath. Soak for 20-30 minutes. Follow the treatment with a hydrating and toning moisturizer for the best effect.

Remember that everyone's skin reacts differently. You should test the products on a less sensitive area before using them.

Memory Bath

Anti-Aging is mostly about the appearance of your skin but if you are like me, your memory can use a bit of a lift now and then too! This bath helps to give your brain a pick me up, lift your spirits, and invigorate your body all while giving your skin a lovely boost.

1/4 cup Ground Mint Leaves

1/4 cup Ground Rosemary

4 tbsp. Ground Basil

4 tbsp. Ground Sage

Blend the powdered herbs and seal them in a clean container with a tightly fitting lid. Add a couple of teaspoons to a warm bath for a lovely and effective aromatic treatment.

You might also blend the herbs and put them in a scrubbing sack or add the herbs to a castile soap base.

While I do add herbs & oils that contain beneficial compounds, I typically do not add color or fragrance to any product designed for damaged skin because additives can cause the irritation to worsen. If you prefer something other than the natural color or scent, you can add your favorite colorant, essential oils, or herbs to the mixture.

Remember that everyone's skin reacts differently. You should test the products on a less sensitive area before using them.

Cellulite Reduction Wrap

This body wrap is a fantastic discovery that actually helps to reduce the appearance of cellulite while hydrating the skin leaving a lush, supple look & feel. We sometimes call this a beach treatment because it makes wearing a bathing suit far less painful

1/4 cup Carrot Juice

1/4 cup Distilled Water

1 tbsp. Wheat Germ Oil

Mix the carrot juice, water, and oils until they are well blended.

2 tbsp. Sea Salt

10 Powdered English Ivy Leaves

Dissolve the sea salt in the liquid solution and then add the English Ivy Powder.

½ cup Powdered Clay

Slowly add the clay powder until the mixture forms a thick paste. If the mixture is too loose for easy application, add a few extra dashes of clay. If the mixture it too solid, add a few extra drops of water.

While I do add herbs & oils that contain beneficial compounds, I typically do not add color or fragrance to any product designed for damaged skin because additives can cause the irritation to worsen. If you prefer something other than the natural color or scent, you can add your favorite colorant, essential oils, or herbs to the mixture.

Pour the completed solution into clean container and seal it tightly.

To use, shake the mixture well and pour ¼ cup into your bath or apply the mixture in a thin, even coat over the area you want to treat.

Allow the mask to work for approximately 20-30 minutes before rinsing your skin.

Follow the treatment with a hydrating and toning moisturizer for the best effect.

Remember that everyone's skin reacts differently. You should test the products on a less sensitive area before using them.

Cleansing Bubble Bath

The basic bubble bath formula helps to clean & hydrate the skin while infusing moisture deep into the surface of the skin. The innate scent of the bath is wonderful & refreshing so this bath is perfect as is.

1/4 cup Liquid Castile Soap

1 tsp. Honey Powder

1 tsp. Hazelnut Oil

1 tbsp. Apricot Kernel Oil

2 tbsp. Coconut Oil

Combine the ingredients and gently mix until they are well blended. Do not whip the mixture since it will foam.

While I do add herbs & oils that contain beneficial compounds, I typically do not add color or fragrance to any product designed for damaged skin because additives can cause the irritation to worsen. If you prefer something other than the natural color or scent, you can add your favorite colorant, essential oils, or herbs to the mixture.

Pour the completed mixture into tightly sealed container.

To use, pour a small amount of the cleanser under the running water as you fill your bath.

Remember that everyone's skin reacts differently. You should test the products on a less sensitive area before using them.

Foaming Bath Gel

I love using this gel in my bath when I know that my skin will be exposed to environmental factors that might contribute to aging. The mixture has an excellent foaming effect that provides a moisturizing, protecting film to your skin. It works especially well for chapped, irritated, or dehydrated skin.

1 tbsp. Grated Beeswax

1/2 cup Jojoba Oil

Heat beeswax and oil in the microwave in a microwave safe dish or in a double broiler until it reaches approximately 90 degrees. Remove the oil from the heat and add

3 tsp. Borax Powder

2 tbsp. Honey

Mix the remaining ingredients with the heated oils until well blended.

While I do add herbs & oils that contain beneficial compounds, I typically do not add color or fragrance to any product designed for damaged skin because additives can cause the irritation to worsen. If you prefer something other than the natural color or scent, you can add your favorite colorant, essential oils, or herbs to the mixture.

Pour the completed mixture into a pump container.

To use, pump one or two squirts into the palm of your hand and apply directly to the skin or into the running bath water.

The oils that remain on the skin after your bath will provide a moisturizing, protective film.

The tub may be slippery and should be cleaned thoroughly after the treatment.

Remember that everyone's skin reacts differently. You should test the products on a less sensitive area before using them.

Pampered Skin Salts

This excellent bath salt works wonders for skin that needs a little pampering. It also works well as a scrub helping to sooth and hydrate the skin while infusing a nice hydrated look.

1 cup Epsom Salts

1 cup Uncooked Oatmeal

2 tsp. Apricot Kernel Oil

1 tsp. Geranium Oil

Combine the dry ingredients in a container.

Pour the oils over the mixture and shake it until the oils are evenly distributed.

While I do add herbs & oils that contain beneficial compounds, I typically do not add color or fragrance to any product designed for damaged skin because additives can cause the irritation to worsen. If you prefer something other than the natural color or scent, you can add your favorite colorant, essential oils, or herbs to the mixture.

To add a fragrance or color sprinkle the desired item over the mixture similar to the way you mixed in the oils.

Shake the salts to distribute the color or fragrance and seal the container tightly.

To use pour approximately ¼ cup in the warm bath water or rub a handful of the mixture over the skin for a nice shower or bath scrub.

Remember that everyone's skin reacts differently. You should test the products on a less sensitive area before using them.

Relaxing Bath Crystals

These crystals are an excellent bath additive that I use whenever I need moisturizing hydration that leaves the skin feeling soft and looking great.

3/4 cup Epsom Salts

1/4 cup Sea Salts

2 tbsp. Chamomile

1 tsp. Hazelnut Oil

1 tsp. Wheat Germ Oil

Crush the chamomile into a fine dust.

Combine the powdered chamomile with the remaining dry ingredients.

Pour the oils over the mixture and shake it until the oils are evenly distributed over the salts.

While I do add herbs & oils that contain beneficial compounds, I typically do not add color or fragrance to any product designed for damaged skin because additives can cause the irritation to worsen. If you prefer something other than the natural color or scent, you can add your favorite colorant, essential oils, or herbs to the mixture.

To add a fragrance or color, sprinkle the desired item over the mixture similar to the way that you mixed in the oils.

Shake the salts to distribute the color or fragrance and seal the container tightly.

To use pour approximately ¼ cup in warm bath water or rub a handful of the mixture over the skin for a nice shower or bath scrub.

Remember that everyone's skin reacts differently. You should test the products on a less sensitive area before using them.

CHAPTER 7

Serums

Healthy skin is not just about cleansing. Healthy skin is about creating the right mixture of cleanliness, hydration, and moisture. Serums & lotions are critical to the success of your skin care regimen.

Some areas of your skin may need additional serums and treatments to help combat the dryness created by other treatments, target specific problems, and reduce the aging process. Serums tend to be lightweight and thinner making applications to the face, neck, and smaller areas easier.

Serums are often oil-based treatments. This helps to maximize the benefits of the serum while minimizing the chance of doing inadvertent damage through the use of additives like thickening agents.

Lotions work much like serums but are traditionally thicker and heavier. While serums work well on the face, lotions tend to be a better choice for the body. Some of the lotions and creams in this guide are suitable for any area of skin. I have included both categories for you to choose the recipe that will work best for you.

Remember that everyone's skin reacts differently. You should test the products on a less sensitive area before using them.

Firming Serum

This is a wonderful massage for the eye and neck oil, especially before bed. It works wonders all over the face if your skin is exceptionally dry.

2 tsp. Olive Oil

2 tsp. Shea Butter

1 tsp. Apricot Kernel Oil

1/2 tsp. Vitamin E Oil

1/2 tsp. Argon Oil

Emulsifier & Thickener as desired

While I do add herbs & oils that contain beneficial compounds, I typically do not add color or fragrance to any product designed for damaged skin because additives can cause the irritation to worsen. If you prefer something other than the natural color or scent, you can add your favorite colorant, essential oils, or herbs to the mixture.

Gently blend the oils in a clean container. Store the mixture in a pump container that allows you to dispense 1 or 2 drops at a time. The oils may separate if allowed to sit so shake the mixture well before each use. Apply an even coat of the oils to the skin in the morning and at night. Do not rinse the mixture from the skin.

Remember that everyone's skin reacts differently. You should test the products on a less sensitive area before using them.

Sensitive Skin Firming Serum

This serum works very well for sensitive skin. It also helps to firm the skin and reduce the puffiness that can make our eyes look tired.

2 tsp. Tamanu Oil

2 tsp. Sunflower Oil

While I do add herbs & oils that contain beneficial compounds, I typically do not add color or fragrance to any product designed for damaged skin because additives can cause the irritation to worsen. If you prefer something other than the natural color or scent, you can add your favorite colorant, essential oils, or herbs to the mixture.

Gently blend the oils in a clean container. Store the mixture in a pump container that allows you to dispense 1 or 2 drops at a time. The oils may separate if allowed to sit so shake the mixture well before each use. Apply an even coat of the oils to the skin in the morning and at night. Do not rinse the mixture from the skin.

Remember that everyone's skin reacts differently. You should test the products on a less sensitive area before using them.

Hydrating Serum

Jojoba is an excellent base for serums since it is close to the skins natural oils and easily absorbed. This is my base facial serum for every day use.

2 tsp. Jojoba Oil

2 tsp. Peanut Oil

1 tsp. Palmarosa Oil

Emulsifier & Thickener as desired

While I do add herbs & oils that contain beneficial compounds, I typically do not add color or fragrance to any product designed for damaged skin because additives can cause the irritation to worsen. If you prefer something other than the natural color or scent, you can add your favorite colorant, essential oils, or herbs to the mixture.

Gently blend the oils in a clean container. Store the mixture in a pump container that allows you to dispense 1 or 2 drops at a time. The oils may separate if allowed to sit so shake the mixture well before each use. Apply an even coat of the oils to the skin in the morning and at night. Do not rinse the mixture from the skin.

Remember that everyone's skin reacts differently. You should test the products on a less sensitive area before using them.

Fine Line Serum

Fine lines are one of my biggest problems. This serum helps to tighten the skin and minimize the appearance of fine lines especially around the eye and mouth area.

2 tsp. Apricot Kernel Oil

2 tsp. Evening Primrose Oil

1 tsp. Grape Seed Oil

Emulsifier & Thickener as desired

While I do add herbs & oils that contain beneficial compounds, I typically do not add color or fragrance to any product designed for damaged skin because additives can cause the irritation to worsen. If you prefer something other than the natural color or scent, you can add your favorite colorant, essential oils, or herbs to the mixture.

Gently blend the oils in a clean container. Store the mixture in a pump container that allows you to dispense 1 or 2 drops at a time. The oils may separate if allowed to sit so shake the mixture well before each use. Apply an even coat of the oils to the skin in the morning and at night. Do not rinse the mixture from the skin.

Remember that everyone's skin reacts differently. You should test the products on a less sensitive area before using them.

Daily Toning Serum

A nice toning serum helps to tighten & refine the appearance of pores while giving the skin a smooth, lustrous appearance.

2 tsp. Sunflower Seed Oil

1/2 tsp. Cypress Oil

1/2 tsp. Hazelnut Oil

Emulsifier & Thickener as desired

While I do add herbs & oils that contain beneficial compounds, I typically do not add color or fragrance to any product designed for damaged skin because additives can cause the irritation to worsen. If you prefer something other than the natural color or scent, you can add your favorite colorant, essential oils, or herbs to the mixture.

Gently blend the oils in a clean container. Store the mixture in a pump container that allows you to dispense 1 or 2 drops at a time. The oils may separate if allowed to sit so shake the mixture well before each use. Apply an even coat of the oils to the skin in the morning and at night. Do not rinse the mixture from the skin.

Remember that everyone's skin reacts differently. You should test the products on a less sensitive area before using them.

Nighttime Toning Gel

This toning gel helps to reduce puffiness, plump the skin and sooth tired eyes all at once. This can be too much for those with especially sensitive skin so do c skin test before use. Aloe tends to leave a shiny residue behind when it dries so this makes a better nighttime treatment.

1 tbsp. Aloe Vera Gel

1 tbsp. Fresh Cucumber juice

1/4 tsp. Geranium Oil

Emulsifier & Thickener as desired

Heat the aloe and cumber juice about 30 seconds on the microwaves high setting or in a double broiler to heat it until the mixture reaches approximately 90 degrees.

Remove the mixture from the heat and allow it to cool slightly until it reaches about 70 degrees.

Stir the oils into the base, mixing until all of the ingredients are well blended.

Store the finished recipe in the refrigerator in a clean container with a tight fitting lid.

While I do add herbs & oils that contain beneficial compounds, I typically do not add color or fragrance to any product designed for damaged skin because additives can cause the irritation to worsen. If you prefer something other than the natural color or scent, you can add your favorite colorant, essential oils, or herbs to the mixture.

The oils may separate if allowed to sit so shake the mixture well before each use. Dab the oils onto the skin that needs treated. Do not rinse the oils from your skin.

Remember that everyone's skin reacts differently. You should test the products on a less sensitive area before using them.

Collagen Building Serum

Collagen loss is one of the most common reasons people seek out anti-aging skin care products. This is a nice serum that helps stimulate collagen production while acting to reduce fine lines & wrinkles.

2 tsp. Hazelnut Oil

1 tsp. Borage Seed Oil

1/2 tsp. Aloe Vera

Emulsifier & Thickener as desired

While I do add herbs & oils that contain beneficial compounds, I typically do not add color or fragrance to any product designed for damaged skin because additives can cause the irritation to worsen. If you prefer something other than the natural color or scent, you can add your favorite colorant, essential oils, or herbs to the mixture.

Gently blend the oils in a clean container. Store the mixture in a pump container that allows you to dispense 1 or 2 drops at a time. The oils may separate if allowed to sit so shake the mixture well before each use. Apply an even coat of the oils to the skin in the morning and at night. Do not rinse the mixture from the skin.

Remember that everyone's skin reacts differently. You should test the products on a less sensitive area before using them.

Acne & Seborrhea Clearing Serum

Even adults can suffer from acne. Seborrhea is actually the most common manifestation in aging skin. This serum helps to reduce the appearance of acne & seborrhea while acting to prevent future outbreaks.

2 tsp. Jojoba Oil

1/4 tsp. Sweet Gale

1/4 tsp. Bayberry

Emulsifier & Thickener as desired

While I do add herbs & oils that contain beneficial compounds, I typically do not add color or fragrance to any product designed for damaged skin because additives can cause the irritation to worsen. If you prefer something other than the natural color or scent, you can add your favorite colorant, essential oils, or herbs to the mixture.

Gently blend the oils in a clean container. Store the mixture in a pump container that allows you to dispense 1 or 2 drops at a time. The oils may separate if allowed to sit so shake the mixture well before each use. Apply an even coat of the oils to the skin in the morning and at night. Do not rinse the mixture from the skin.

Remember that everyone's skin reacts differently. You should test the products on a less sensitive area before using them.

Seborrhea Serum

This wonderful serum helps to reduce the appearance of both seborrhea and acne while hydrating the skin and combating fine lines. It is the first serum I whip up when someone has seborrhea.

1 tsp. Jojoba Oil

1 tsp. Argan Oil

1 tsp. Immortelle Oil

2 tsp. Sea Buckthorn Oil

Emulsifier & Thickener as desired

While I do add herbs & oils that contain beneficial compounds, I typically do not add color or fragrance to any product designed for damaged skin because additives can cause the irritation to worsen. If you prefer something other than the natural color or scent, you can add your favorite colorant, essential oils, or herbs to the mixture.

Gently blend the oils in a clean container. Store the mixture in a pump container that allows you to dispense 1 or 2 drops at a time. The oils may separate if allowed to sit so shake the mixture well before each use. Apply an even coat of the oils to the skin in the morning and at night. Do not rinse the mixture from the skin.

Remember that everyone's skin reacts differently. You should test the products on a less sensitive area before using them.

Pore Reduction Serum

One of the hardest parts of managing aging skin is getting the wrinkle reduction action while helping to reduce enlarged pores. This is a nice serum for reducing the appearance of pores while maximizing the anti-aging actions of other treatments.

2 tsp. Rosewater

1/4 tsp. Lemongrass Oil

5 drops Patchouli Oil

While I do add herbs & oils that contain beneficial compounds, I typically do not add color or fragrance to any product designed for damaged skin because additives can cause the irritation to worsen. If you prefer something other than the natural color or scent, you can add your favorite colorant, essential oils, or herbs to the mixture.

Gently blend the oils in a clean container. Store the mixture in a pump container that allows you to dispense 1 or 2 drops at a time. The oils may separate if allowed to sit so shake the mixture well before each use. Apply an even coat of the oils to the skin in the morning and at night. Do not rinse the mixture from the skin.

Remember that everyone's skin reacts differently. You should test the products on a less sensitive area before using them.

Daily Dark Spot Reduction Serum

Sometimes aging can leave marks. When these marks are pigmentation spots, also known as age spots, you can help to fade them with the proper treatments. This is one of my favorites and best of all it works on freckles too!

2 tsp. Kukui Nut Oil

1 tsp. Powdered Gotu Kola

1/2 tsp. Vitamin E Oil

1/2 tsp. Magnolia Oil

Emulsifier & Thickener as desired

While I do add herbs & oils that contain beneficial compounds, I typically do not add color or fragrance to any product designed for damaged skin because additives can cause the irritation to worsen. If you prefer something other than the natural color or scent, you can add your favorite colorant, essential oils, or herbs to the mixture.

Gently blend the oils in a clean container. Store the mixture in a pump container that allows you to dispense 1 or 2 drops at a time. The oils may separate if allowed to sit so shake the mixture well before each use. Dab the oils onto areas with dark pigmentation. Allow the oils to absorb naturally. Do not rinse the oils from your skin. The fading action is most pronounced when the oils are applied at least 3 times a day and not diluted with other lotions or make up.

Remember that everyone's skin reacts differently. You should test the products on a less sensitive area before using them.

Nighttime Spot Reduction Gel

This gel is a nice alternative age spot reducing cream. It works best as a nighttime treatment because the gel tends to be a little shiny when it dries. This may not be as powerful as the Daily Dark Spot Reduction Serum but it also tends to be less irritating for those with sensitive skin.

2 tsp. Aloe Vera Gel

2 tsp. Powdered Asphodelus

While I do add herbs & oils that contain beneficial compounds, I typically do not add color or fragrance to any product designed for damaged skin because additives can cause the irritation to worsen. If you prefer something other than the natural color or scent, you can add your favorite colorant, essential oils, or herbs to the mixture.

Gently blend the oils in a clean container. Store the mixture in a pump container that allows you to dispense 1 or 2 drops at a time. The oils may separate if allowed to sit so shake the mixture well before each use. Dab the oils onto areas with dark pigmentation. Allow the oils to absorb naturally. Do not rinse the oils from your skin. The fading action is most pronounced when the oils are applied at least 3 times a day and not diluted with other lotions or make up.

Remember that everyone's skin reacts differently. You should test the products on a less sensitive area before using them.

CHAPTER 8

Lotions and Creams

Once you have clean and healthy looking skin, the next important focus to reducing the aging process is moisture. Your skin needs moisture to look its best. These lotions tend to work well on the body since they contain ingredients that help to expand the products cutting down on the concentration, costs, and effects.

The basic ingredients in moisturizing products are oil and water. Most creams also contain an emulsifier.

An emulsifier is a waxy substance that aids in keeping oil and water from separating. If you choose not to use an emulsifier, the creams and lotions you create will provide the same benefits but the components may separate when the product is left to sit. To correct this separation, shake the skin care product well before applying. This will serve to combine the ingredients and is an effective solution if you don't want an emulsifier in your mixture.

I typically do not use an emulsifier in my anti-aging recipes. Since environmental factors contribute heavily to aging, I try to minimize the excess compounds that I include in my recipes.

I do sometimes use a thickening agent to help make the lotions easier to apply so some of the recipes already contain a beneficial thickening agent. Before modifying the recipe to include a thickening agent or an emulsifier, you should remember that these ingredients also have an affect on the skin.

Before you decide which recipes are right for you, you must determine what type of skin you have. There are four basic types of skin: normal, dry, oily, and combination.

Dry skin does not always occur when skin is deprived of oils. It often occurs when water is lacking in the skin. This means that for those of us with dry skin, hydrating the skin from the inside as well as the out can go a long way toward curing our most basic skin problems. Dry skin can become very irritated and unattractive.

Proper care and hydration can cure the most common and basic dry skin problems. If you have allowed the problem to become excessive or if you suffer from a specific skin disorder, it is best to seek the input of your dermatologist before trying any self-created products as some skin disorders can actually be aggravated by the use of the wrong product.

Oily skin is a surplus of oil on the surface of the skin as well as a build up of oils below the surface that can result in unsightly eruptions and irritation. You will want to limit the amount of oils you utilize if your skin tends towards oily. Healthy skin has the ability to generate enough oils on its own and one of the focuses of your regimen will be to nourish and care for your skin while limiting the amount of external oil you apply.

There is a very simple method of determining your skin type. Wash your face with your favorite basic cleanser. Pat your skin dry and do not apply any products to your skin. After a couple of hours take a clean cloth or tissue paper and blot your forehead, nose and cheeks. Use a new cloth for each area of the skin. If oily spots appear on the cloth, your skin could be considered oily. If there is only a small amount of oil on the cloths, your skin is probably normal. If no oil appears on any of the cloths, your skin is likely dry.

Skin can change for a variety of reasons: aging changes the oil levels in your skin, as do climatic conditions and hormone levels. You may want to test your skin during a variety of conditions to determine what products may benefit you the most during what times of the month or year.

These recipes are ones that I use for lotions and creams that will be primarily applied to the body. Serums tend to be my go to option for the face and neck area. You should consider which ones will best suit your facial and body care needs and then choose the serum or lotion recipe that will work best for you.

Remember that everyone's skin reacts differently. You should test the products on a less sensitive area before using them.

Age Defying Lotion

This is an effective lotion for the body. It infuses the skin with various anti-aging, toning and emollient components while helping to reduce irritants that may cause skin problems.

1 tbsp. Crushed Fennel Seeds

1/4 cup Distilled Water

Heat the water until it reaches a light boil. Pour the boiling water over the fennel seeds and allow the mixture to soak overnight. Drain the seeds from the liquid and discard the seeds. The liquid will act as the base for your recipe.

2 tbsp. Grated Beeswax

1 tbsp. Aloe Vera Gel

1 tsp. Vitamin E oil

1 tbsp. Jojoba Oil

Combine beeswax and oils in a microwave safe dish and heat on medium for approximately 25 seconds or use a double boiler to bring the mixture to about 90 degrees.

Remove the mixture from the heat, stir it well and set it aside to cool until it reaches about 70 degrees.

2 tbsp. Aluminum Sulfate

3 tbsp. Witch Hazel

3 tbsp. Orange Flower Water

Emulsifier & Thickener as desired

Use only *USP Grade for Cosmetic Use* aluminum sulfates.

Use only plastic or ceramic pans and utensils since aluminum sulfate can react with metals.

Dissolve the aluminum sulfate in the witch hazel and orange flower water.

Add the fennel seed liquid and stir the mixture until it is well blended.

Slowly pour the liquid solution into the oil base stirring well.

The mixture will foam slightly as you stir.

The product will have its own natural scent and color, but if you desire a specific color to suit your needs or an aromatherapy benefit you may add your favorite colorant or essential oils to the recipe. While I do add herbs & oils that contain beneficial compounds, I typically do not add color or fragrance to any product designed for damaged skin because additives can cause the irritation to worsen.

Spoon the finished lotion into a clean container with a tight fitting lid. Allow the mixture to cool completely before use.

Massage the lotion in to the skin twice daily for the most beneficial results.

Remember that everyone's skin reacts differently. You should test the products on a less sensitive area before using them.

Skin Smoothing Lotion

This lovely light lotion is great for year round care. The corn flour provides a silky texture to the lotion that leaves the skin feeling supple and smooth while the natural humectants qualities of the glycerin attract moisture to provide a softening quality.

3 tbsp. Glycerin

3 tbsp. Corn Flour (cornstarch powder)

1/4 cup Rose Water

1/4 cup Distilled Water

Emulsifier & Thickener as desired

Mix all of the ingredients in a microwave safe dish and heat for approximately 1 minute until the mixture just begins to boil.   Stir the mixture every 20-25 seconds during heating. You may also heat the mixture to a light boil in a double broiler.

The product will have its own natural scent and color, but if you desire a specific color to suit your needs or an aromatherapy benefit you may add your favorite colorant or essential oils to the recipe. While I do add herbs & oils that contain beneficial compounds, I typically do not add color or fragrance to any product designed for damaged skin because additives can cause the irritation to worsen. If you prefer something other than the natural color or scent, you can add your favorite colorant, essential oils, or herbs to the mixture.

Pour the finished lotion into a clean container and seal it tightly. Allow the lotion to cool completely before use.

To use pump or pour a small amount into the palm of your hand and massage gently into the skin. This lotion is more gel like so you will need to use care until you learn to manage the application.

Remember that everyone's skin reacts differently. You should test the products on a less sensitive area before using them.

Pear Lotion for Red Blotchy Skin

This is a great treatment to use anytime environmental factors create havoc with your skin. It also helps to reduce the red, flaky skin associated with seborrhea while providing essential hydration and nourishment. I love the soft scent of the pears, but you could use other fruits that contain sorbitol such as apples, cherries, plums or berries. Sorbitol is a natural humectant that attracts moisture and provides a smooth texture to the skin.

2 tbsp. Grated Beeswax

2 tbsp. Jojoba Oil

1/4 cup Sesame Seed Oil

1/4 cup Juice (pear, apple, cherry, plum or berry)

2 tbsp. Witch Hazel

1/4 tsp. Borax Powder

Emulsifier & Thickener as desired

Place the beeswax and oils in a microwave safe dish and heat on medium approximately 25 seconds or use a double broiler to liquefy the mixture bringing it to approximately 90 degrees Fahrenheit. Remove the mixture from the heat and allow it to cool to approximately 70 degrees.

Combine the remaining ingredients in another dish.

Heat the witch hazel mixture unit it is hot but not boiling - approximately 35 seconds on medium heat.

Pour the juice mixture into the oil mixture and stir until well blended.

I love the natural smells and colors of this recipe and can alter the final product by changing the type of juice I use.

While I do add herbs & oils that contain beneficial compounds, I typically do not add color or fragrance to any product designed for damaged skin because additives can cause the irritation to worsen. If you prefer something other than the natural color or scent, you can add your favorite colorant, essential oils, or herbs to the mixture.

Allow the recipe to cool before use. The mixture will thicken as it cools.

Remember that everyone's skin reacts differently. You should test the products on a less sensitive area before using them.

Deep Hydration Lotion

Skin doesn't just need moisture on the surface it needs moisture deep down. Hydrating washes, lotions and treatments provide the benefit of total moisture infusion. This lotion is great for deep hydration and can be used daily to provide a supple, healthy appearance to skin.

2 tbsp. Dried Chamomile Leaves

1/2 cup Distilled Water

Heat the water until it is just boiling. Remove the water from the heat and pour it over the chamomile leaves. Allow the mixture to steep at least 6 hours until a darker tea is created. Strain the leaves from the tea and discard them. The liquid will act as your lotion base. Add

1 tsp. Baking Soda

3 tbsp. Glycerin

Combine the baking soda and glycerin with the chamomile water in c microwave safe dish. Heat on medium until the mixture just reaches boiling approximately 1 minute.

3 tbsp. Stearic Acid Powder

1/4 cup Jojoba Oil

Emulsifier & Thickener as desired

In another dish, combine the oils and stearic acid. Heat them on mecium in the microwave for about 30 seconds until the liquid runs clear or in a double broiler until the mixture reaches about 90 degrees.

½ cup Carrot Juice

Add the carrot juice to the chamomile tea mixture and stir gently.

Slowly pour the chamomile mixture into the oil base.

The mixture will foam as it is mixed.

Stir gently to combine all of the ingredients.

Allow mixture to cool.

The mixture will have a pretty golden orange color and a delicate fragrance. If you desire a personalized fragrance or color, you may add food coloring or your favorite essential oils to the mixture as it cools. While I do add herbs & oils that contain beneficial compounds, I typically do not add color or fragrance to any product designed for damaged skin because additives can cause the irritation to worsen. If you prefer something other than the natural color or scent, you can add your favorite colorant, essential oils, or herbs to the mixture.

Pour the lotion into a clean container and allow it to cool completely.

The mixture will thicken as it stands. Tightly seal the container.

This lotion will not keep as long as some others because of the juices. It may be stored in the refrigerator to lengthen the shelf life.

Remember that everyone's skin reacts differently. You should test the products on a less sensitive area before using them.

Daily Lotion

Daily hydration is essential for healthy, youthful looking skin. This is a nice general lotion for every day use.

1/4 cup Almond Oil

1/8 cup Stearic Acid Powder

1 tbsp. Hazelnut Oil

1/4 cup Pear Juice

1/4 cup Carrot Juice

1 tsp. Baking Soda

2-3 drops Tincture of Benzoin

Emulsifier & Thickener as desired

Heat the almond oil, stearic acid and hazelnut oil in the microwave on medium heat until mixture turns golden and foamy – approximately 35 seconds. You can also heat the mixture in a double broiler to approximately 90 degrees.

Remove the oils from the heat and set them aside to cool to about 70 degrees.

Combine remaining ingredients in another dish.

Whip the mixture with a whisk or in a blender until it foams slightly and all ingredients are well blended.

While I do add herbs & oils that contain beneficial compounds, I typically do not add color or fragrance to any product designed for damaged skin because additives can cause the irritation to worsen. If you prefer something other than the natural color or scent, you can add your favorite colorant, essential oils, or herbs to the mixture.

Pour the lotion into a clean container and allow it to cool. The lotion will thicken as it cools.

Remember that everyone's skin reacts differently. You should test the products on a less sensitive area before using them.

Glowing Daily Lotion

There are many products on the market that provide an unnatural glow to the skin. These products contain everything from crystals to metal. This fantastic lotion will allow your skins natural glow to shine through without creating additional irritation that may lead to irritation or aging. I love to use this lotion in the summer months when my skin needs nourishment and I can show off the natural glow that is a part of my skin.

2 tbsp. Grated Beeswax

1 tbsp. Palma Rosa Oil

Place the beeswax in a microwave safe dish and heat on medium approximately 25 seconds or use a double broiler to melt the beeswax bringing it to about 90 degrees. Remove the beeswax from the heat and add

1/4 cup Sea Buckthorn

1/4 tsp. Borax Powder

Slowly add the borax mixture to the beeswax syrup.

1/4 cup Aloe Vera Gel

Emulsifier & Thickener as desired

Add the aloe vera gel to the base mixture and blend the ingredients until they are well mixed.

While I do add herbs & oils that contain beneficial compounds, I typically do not add color or fragrance to any product designed for damaged skin because additives can cause the irritation to worsen. If you prefer something other than the natural color or scent, you can add your favorite colorant, essential oils, or herbs to the mixture.

Pour the lotion into a clean container and allow it to cool completely.

The mixture will thicken as it stands. Tightly seal the container.

Remember that everyone's skin reacts differently. You should test the products on a less sensitive area before using them.

Nourishing Daily Lotion

Wel-nourished skin is beautiful skin. This lotion is full of compounds that are vital for nourished, healthy skin and is light enough for every day use.

1/2 cup Apricot Kernel Oil

1 tbsp. Grated Beeswax

1 tbsp. Almond Oil

Combine the oils and beeswax in a microwave safe dish and heat on medium for about 25 seconds or until the liquids melt to a consistency similar to syrup. You can also use a double broiler to heat the oils & wax to approximately 90 degrees.

Remove the mixture from the heat and set it aside to cool slightly until it reaches approximately 70 degrees Fahrenheit. Add

1/4 tsp. Borax Powder

1/2 cup Distilled Water

Emulsifier & Thickener as desired

Dissolve the borax powder in the water. You may need to heat the water slightly to help dissolve the crystals.

Slowly add the borax mixture to the beeswax syrup.

You should use a wire whisk or a blender to ensure the ingredients are well mixed.

While I do add herbs & oils that contain beneficial compounds, I typically do not add color or fragrance to any product designed for damaged or sensitive skin because additives can cause the irritation to worsen. If you prefer something other than the natural color or scent, you can add your favorite colorant, essential oils, or herbs to the mixture.

Spoon the finished liquid into a clean container with a tight fitting lid. Allow the mixture to cool completely before use.

Massage the lotion in to the skin twice daily for the most beneficial results.

Remember that everyone's skin reacts differently. You should test the products on a less sensitive area before using them.

Deep Moisturizing Cream

This is a deep penetrating cream that I use all over but truly love after a rough skin exfoliation. Beyond the penetration, the treatment leaves a protective film on the skin that helps to prevent drying. We like to make a heat pack out of this during the winter months by applying a thicker layer of the cream and then covering the treated area with plastic to let the oils really penetrate the skin.

1/2 cup Sesame Oil

1/4 cup Wheat Germ Oil

2 tbsp. Grated Beeswax

2 tbsp. Coconut Oil

Emulsifier & Thickener as desired

Heat the oils and beeswax for approximately 25 seconds on medium in the microwave or until they form a thick syrup. You an also heat the ingredients to approximately 90 degrees Fahrenheit using a double broiler.

Remove the mixture from the heat and allow it to cool, stirring occasionally to prevent separation during the cooling stage.

While I do add herbs & oils that contain beneficial compounds, I typically do not add color or fragrance to any product designed for damaged skin because additives can cause the irritation to worsen. If you prefer something other than the natural color or scent, you can add your favorite colorant, essential oils, or herbs to the mixture.

Store the lotion in a clean container with a tight fitting lid.

To use, apply the lotion directly to the desired area and massage gently.

For a deeper conditioning action, heat the mixture slightly under warm water and apply a thick coat to desired areas. Cover the areas with saran wrap or a plastic bag and allow the mixture to penetrate the skin for 10-15 minutes.

Wipe remaining lotion from skin, but do not rinse the protective film off the skin.

Remember that everyone's skin reacts differently. You should test the products on a less sensitive area before using them.

Protective Lotion

This lotion provides extra skin protection ingredients. I like to use this whenever I have been using a lot specialized treatments that make my skin extra dry & sensitive. The beeswax and oils form a protective layer on the skin making it difficult for dirt and harmful chemicals to cause further damage. This is a great lotion year round for normal to dry skin.

2 tbsp. Grated Beeswax

1/4 tsp. Borax Powder

1/4 cup Jojoba Oil

1/4 cup Tincture of Benzoin

1/4 cup Distilled Water

Emulsifier & Thickener as desired

Place the beeswax, honey and oil in a microwave safe dish and heat on medium approximately 25 seconds or use a double broiler to liquefy the ingredients bringing them to approximately 90 degrees Fahrenheit.

Remove the mixture from the microwave and set aside to cool slightly until it reaches about 70 degrees.

Dissolve the borax powder in the water and heat it until it is just boiling.

Slowly pour the borax solution into the oil and beeswax mixture.

Whip the mixture with a whisk or in a blender until it foams slightly and all ingredients are well blended.

While I do add herbs & oils that contain beneficial compounds, I typically do not add color or fragrance to any product designed for damaged skin because additives can cause the irritation to worsen. If you prefer something other than the natural color or scent, you can add your favorite colorant, essential oils, or herbs to the mixture.

Pour the lotion into a clean container and allow it to cool.   The lotion will thicken as it cools.

Remember that everyone's skin reacts differently. You should test the products on a less sensitive area before using them.

Firming Night Lotion

I like to make nighttime treatments a bit more powerful since the lotion can stay on the skin for hours at a time without being disturbed. This nutritive, oil based lotion permeates the skin and helps you wake up with beautiful, supple skin!

2 tbsp. Coconut Oil

2 tbsp. Almond Oil

2 tsp. Apricot Kernel Oil

1 tsp. Vitamin E Oil

6 tbsp. Aloe Vera Gel

Emulsifier & Thickener as desired

Combine all of the oils in a microwave safe dish and heat on medium approximately 25 seconds or use a double broiler to bring the oils to about 70 degrees.

Remove the mixture from the microwave and pour it into the aloe vera gel.

Whip the mixture with a whisk or in a blender until it foams slightly and all of the ingredients are well blended.

While I do add herbs & oils that contain beneficial compounds, I typically do not add color or fragrance to any product designed for damaged skin because additives can cause the irritation to worsen. If you prefer something other than the natural color or scent, you can add your favorite colorant, essential oils, or herbs to the mixture.

Pour the lotion into a clean container and allow it to cool. The lotion will thicken as it cools.

Remember that everyone's skin reacts differently. You should test the products on a less sensitive area before using them.

Skin Toning Lotion

At times, I want an all over body toning product and combining a moisture infusing lotion with the benefits of a toning action really saves time. This great lotion provides a fresh clean feel while delivering toning agents to my skin.

2 tbsp. Apricot Kernel Oil

1 tbsp. Hazelnut Oil

2 tbsp. Wheat Germ Oil

Heat the oils for approximately 25 seconds on medium heat in the microwave or to about 70 degrees using a double broiler. Remove the oils from the heat.

1/4 cup Witch Hazel

2 tbsp. Rosewater

1/4 cup Stearic Acid Powder

Emulsifier & Thickener as desired

Dissolve the powders in the witch hazel & rosewater. Slowly pour the liquid into the oil base, stirring well.

While I do add herbs & oils that contain beneficial compounds, I typically do not add color or fragrance to any product designed for damaged or sensitive skin because additives can cause the irritation to worsen. If you prefer something other than the natural color or scent, you can add your favorite colorant, essential oils, or herbs to the mixture.

Pour the lotion into a clean container and allow it to cool. The lotion will thicken as it cools.

Remember that everyone's skin reacts differently. You should test the products on a less sensitive area before using them.

CHAPTER 9

Mineral Makeup

Once your skin is clean, treated, and hydrated you may want to add makeup to enhance your overall appearance. Selecting a makeup can be a tough decision for those whose skin is really beginning to show signs of aging. You certainly do not want to select a makeup that is going to undo all that you have achieved through selective skin treatments. One solution that's becoming a popular choice among women of all ages is mineral makeup.

Mineral make up has been used for hundreds, even thousands of years across the globe. Over the last few years, interest in this natural skin colorant has undergone a tremendous boost. Many companies have developed lines of mineral makeup. Each touts the benefits of their line over the next. Whether one is better than another is a matter of opinion and I am not going to express mine here!

What I am going to do is tell you a few of the benefits all of these lines (and homemade mineral makeup) offer to you. Then, I will show you the recipe that I use to make mineral make up at home for myself, my daughter, my daughter's classmates and friends and even some of my friends and family. I like the make up that I make at home, love that I can feel comfortable having 'girl's day' with my 9 year old and her friends without worrying that I am ruining their skin, and especially love that it costs me pennies to make a years supply of makeup for everyone!

Mineral makeup is a wholly natural make up product created mostly from powdered minerals. The benefits of mineral make up are numerous but the most influential factor to most people is that it is 100% natural.

BENEFITS:

Mineral makeup is made from zinc and titanium dioxide so it is a natural sunscreen. Depending on how much you use SPF can range from 10 to 20.

Mineral makeup is typically water resistant. That is not to say waterproof but it does last much better while swimming or during water sports than many other make up products.

Mineral makeup is long-lasting, bearing up better to long days, outdoor activity, and even naps than more traditional make up products.

Mineral makeup contains ingredients that have special properties of their own. In addition to offering a natural sunscreen, you receive the side-benefits of each ingredient. If you look at the recipe for mineral base, you will see that zinc oxide is a main component. Zinc oxide has natural anti-inflammatory properties so the make up you make with zinc oxide will too!

When applied correctly, the coverage offered by mineral make up is lightweight and complete. This makes it perfect for all skin types – from young to old, oily to dry and everything in between.

Mineral make up is non-comedogenic and (unless you add oils to the recipe) oil free! This means it is less harmful and irritating to your skin. Some makers say it is so clean you can even sleep in it!

Mineral make up is all-natural and the ingredients (unless you add oils to the recipe) do not go bad. That means you do not have to add any preservatives to the mix making it healthier and more natural than the next makeup!

Mineral make up is fast and easy to apply.

Mineral make up is VERY inexpensive to make at home.

Base or Foundation

Base or foundation is applied all over the face to create a smooth texture, even skin tone, and flawless finish.

4 tsp. Micronized Titanium Dioxide

1 1/2 tsp. Bismuth Oxychloride

2 tsp. Zinc Oxide – Low Micron

1/2 tsp. Magnesium Stearate

Mix base ingredients by blending well. You can use a mortar / pestle, metal spoon and bowl, or food processor to blend the ingredients.

Slowly add the pigment colorant to the mix.

+/- to preference

1/4 tsp. Yellow Iron Oxide

Pinch Brown Iron Oxide

Pinch Red Iron Oxide

1/2 tsp. Sericite Mica - matte or translucent finish to suit final goals

You can change the tint of the final product to suit your skin tone and color preferences.

For darker shades, add more of any of the iron oxides.

For lighter shades, add more titanium dioxide or some sericite mica.

Some people have reported that Bismuth Oxychloride causes irritation and redness. If you have sensitive skin or develop a reaction to the recipe, you may try using less or no Bismuth Oxychloride in your recipe.

You might want to experiment with different color additives to correct or address certain problems. You could start with:

Yellow Oxide brightens dull complexions and counteracts redness.

Chromium Oxide Green counters redness from seborrhea, acne, or irritated skin.

Ultramarine Violet counters yellow or sallow skin tones; minimizes yellowish bruises.

Ultramarine Blue counters orange tones that may result from sunless tanning products.

LIQUID APPLICATION – some people prefer a bit more moisture in their makeup or like a liquid application more than a dry application. We make a liquid application by adding the powder mixture to our preferred moisturizer. The consistency of the liquid application is entirely a matter of preference. You will want to experiment by slowly adding the mineral mixture to your favorite moisturizer until you achieve the consistency and coverage amount you desire. The consistency ranges from full coverage matt to a lightweight tinted moisturizer.

Mineral Veil – Finish Powder

Mineral Veil is also called a finish powder and gives the face a translucent glow. It is applied on top of all other makeup.

3 tsp. Sericite Mica – Matte

1 tsp. Corn Starch

1/2 tsp. Boron Nitrate

1/2 tsp. Magnesium Stearate

Mix base ingredients by blending well. You can use a mortar / pestle, metal spoon and bowl, or food processor to blend the ingredients.

Slowly add the pigment colorant to the mix.

+/- to preference

Pinch Yellow Iron Oxide

Pinch Pink

Pinch Brown Iron Oxide

You can change the tint of the final product to suit your skin tone and color preferences.

For darker shades, add more of any of the iron oxides.

For lighter shades, add more Corn Starch.

Concealer

A concealer is similar to a foundation in composition with a few simple modifications. Concealer tends to be a couple of shades lighter than your foundation, provides more coverage and is more matte in finish.

1/2 tbsp   . Micronized Titanium Dioxide

1/2 tbsp. Seracite Mica – Matte

1/4 tbsp. Magnesium Stearate

Mix base ingredients by blending well. You can use a mortar / pestle, metal spoon and bowl, or food processor to blend the ingredients.

Slowly add the pigment colorant to the mix.

+/- to preference

1/16 tbsp. Yellow Iron Oxide

Pinch Red or Orange Iron Oxide

You can change the tint of the final product to suit your skin tone and color preferences.

For darker shades, add more of any of the iron oxides.

For lighter shades, add more titanium dioxide or some sericite mica.

You might want to experiment with different color additives to correct or address certain problems. You could start with:

Yellow Oxide brightens dull complexions or counteracts redness.

Chromium Green counters redness from seborrhea, acne, or irritated skin.

Ultramarine Violet counters yellow or sallow skin tones; minimizes yellowish bruises.

Ultramarine Blue counters orange tones that may result from sunless tanning products.

LIQUID APPLICATION - Some people prefer a bit more moisture in their makeup or like a liquid application more than a dry application. We make a liquid application by adding the powder mixture to our preferred moisturizer. The consistency of the liquid application is entirely a matter of preference. You will want to experiment by slowly adding the powder mixture to your favorite moisturizer until you achieve the consistency and coverage amount you desire.

Concealer often needs to be a bit heavier in weight. To create a heavier blend, you may want to try adding more mineral to the moisturizer or use a very heavy moisturizer as the base.

APPLICATION – DRY - To apply concealer in dry or powder form, first apply your foundation then use a small brush to apply the concealer directly to problem areas. Use a larger "Kabuki" brush to blend.

APPLICATION – WET - To apply concealer wet, put a small amount in the palm of your hand, add a small amount of water or moisturizer as desired, and apply with a brush or a sponge to problem areas. By applying wet, you can target larger problem areas. Allow concealer to dry after application. Apply powdered foundation over the concealer to blend and finish.

Bronzer

A bronzer gives extra color where the sun hits the face. The sun leaves a bronze or rosy hue behind. The bronzer gives you the ability to infuse a fresh, healthy glow to your skin without the dangers of spending the day in the sun.

2 tsp. Micronized Titanium Dioxide

1/3 tsp. Magnesium Stearate

Mix base ingredients by blending well. You can use a mortar / pestle, metal spoon and bowl, or food processor to blend the ingredients.

Slowly add the pigment colorant to the mix.

+/- to preference

1/2 tsp. Yellow Iron Oxide

1/2 tsp. Brown Iron Oxide

1/2 tsp. Red Iron Oxide

1 tsp. Sericite Mica – pearl finish

1/2 tsp. Bronze mica

You can change the tint of the final product to suit your skin tone and color preferences.

For darker shades, add more of any of the iron oxides.

For lighter shades, add more titanium dioxide or sericite mica.

Eye Shadow

Eye Shadow is used to give extra attention to the eyes.

1 tbsp. Micronized Titanium Dioxide

1/2 tsp. Magnesium Stearate

1 tsp. Sericite Mica – Pearl or Matte as preferred

Pearl Sericite will give you a shimmer effect eye shadow

Matte Sericite will give you a low luster eye shadow

Mix base ingredients by blending well. You can use a mortar / pestle, metal spoon and bowl, or food processor to blend the ingredients.

Slowly add the pigment colorant to the mix.

+/- to preference

1/2 tsp. Iron Oxide color of your choice

Start with ½ tsp and increase until desired color is obtained

We enjoy mixing multiple colors to attain a shadow that is specific to us. If you custom mix your shadow to your personal preference – DO NOT forget to write down what you did so you can repeat it later.

You can change the tint of the final product to suit your skin tone and color preferences.

For darker shades, add more of any of the iron oxides.

For lighter shades, add more titanium dioxide or some sericite mica.

Blush

Blush is used to accent the cheekbones and provide a healthy color to the face.

2 3/4 tsp. Sericite Mica

1/4 tsp. Micronized Titanium Dioxide

1/16 tsp. Arrowroot Powder

Mix base ingredients by blending well. You can use a mortar / pestle, metal spoon and bowl, or food processor to blend the ingredients.

Slowly add the pigment colorant to the mix.

+/- to preference

1/16 tsp. Red Iron Oxide

Start with 1/16 tsp and increase until desired color is obtained

We enjoy mixing multiple colors to attain a shadow that is specific to us. If you custom mix your shadow to your personal preference – DO NOT forget to write down what you did so you can repeat it later.

CHAPTER 10

Natural Ingredients

The barks, flowers, leaves and roots that have been used for centuries as traditional supplements are still easily obtainable from health food stores, organic growers, and even in the wild. Many of plants used in traditional supplements are also easy to grow. Whether you have a windowsill garden or acreage waiting to be farmed, you can selectively grow, harvest, and process many of the traditional supplements successfully used for thousands of years to treat common ailments.

There are numerous ways of using plant products as supplements. You can use plant products as a drink, flavoring, culinary seasoning, aromatherapy treatment, and so forth. Nearly any supplement preparation you purchase at the store can be made from scratch using plant products. There are numerous natural product recipe guides available, including my Green & Natural book series that include simple recipes that you can create to replace almost every supplement that you use. You can also create your own custom preparations using the plants detailed in the compendium.

The first step in making natural supplements is to know the type of supplements that you need. The second step is to obtain the plant parts that you will use in the creation of the supplements. Most people quickly decide that they want to create their own supplements starting at the beginning. That means growing their own plants to harvest, process, and use.

Each type of flower, herb, shrub, or tree will need a slightly different environment and handling for optimal growth. Propagation of plants is another entire subject that cannot be completely addressed here. If you are interested in propagating many types of plants using different methods, you should obtain a guide to help you along the way. Seed propagation is among the most common ways to get a garden started so we will illustrate how easily you can cultivate your own supplement garden from seeds.

The first step in creating your supplement garden is to decide what plants you want to include. The compendium provides details about plants that have traditionally been used as supplements to address common conditions. You should compile a list of your preferred plants from the pages of the compendium.

As a starting organic grower, you will want to narrow the list to include those plants that fit within your climate and the space that you have available for growing.

You will want to consider the growth patterns of the plants you select for your supplement garden. Planning the types of plants included in the garden helps to ensure that you have an adequate harvest during each season and that you do not need to replace exhausted plants. The two most common classifications of plants you will encounter are the annual and the perennial.

Some plants are annual plants. An annual plant is one that completes its entire life cycle in one year and then dies. Annuals usually grow quickly. When growing annuals for supplement use, you can harvest the entire plant each season. You will start the next season with a new plant. You can even harvest the seeds and process them yourself for next year.

If you live in a warmer climate, you should remember that a plant that is considered an annual in most regions might actually be a perennial in your area. You will want to confirm how the particular plants you select grow in your region before completely harvesting it in case the plant might yield more growth.

A perennial plant is a plant that continues to grow year after year. Many of the plants in the compendium are perennial plants. In some regions, perennial plants will simply continue to grow, going through slower and faster cycles of growth. In other regions, perennial plants may enter a period of dormancy followed by a period of new growth. You will usually not want to harvest all of the parts of a perennial plant. You should take only as much as you need from the plant and leave the rest so that the plant can continue to grow, regularly producing new crops for you to use.

Once you have a compiled a listing of the plants that you want to cultivate, you can obtain seedlings from a grower or purchase seeds from a reputable supplier. Most home supplement growers prefer to grow their plants from seeds.

The cost of growing a plant from seed is often much lower than the cost of purchasing seedlings or adult plants. In addition, when you grow a plant yourself, you know the exact history of the plant. You can feel confident that no chemicals were used during the growing process and that the plant you will be using as a supplement is healthy.

If you are growing from seed, you will need to gather a few items.

Seeds
Potting Medium
Coverage
Light Source

You will want to obtain containers that are safe for plant growth. There are many available growing containers. All natural, biodegradable plant starters are among the most environmentally friendly and chemical free options. These tend to be more costly than some other options and may not be worthwhile if you are keeping the mature plants indoors instead of transferring them to an outside space. There is a wide variety of seeding options available and you should select the one that will be most useful in your garden plant. The biggest consideration when selecting a container for supplement growing is to ensure that they are not made of a plastic product that can degrade and cause damage to your plants or cause the plant to ingest chemicals that will then contaminate any products you make from that plant.

The container you select should allow for water drainage. The commercially sold planting cups are usually created with a drainage feature. If you are making your own planting cups, you will want to put a few small holes in the bottom to allow excess water to drain away from the roots.

You will need to purchase pre-mixed seeding medium or harvest your own from a nutrient rich area of your yard. If you are a regular gardener, you know where the best potting soil can be found. If you are a beginner, purchasing pre-mixed organic seeding mix is typically a better choice. Seeding mix should be light enough to allow for good air circulation but not so light that it creates an unsustainable rooting medium for the plants if you are moving them outdoors.

Fill each of your seed cups ¾ of the way full with seeding mix. Gently tap or press the soil to ensure there are no air pockets. Air pockets can cause the seed to drop too deeply into the soil and may make it difficult for young roots to find sufficient nutrients. A young root that encounters an air pocket is likely to wither and die weakening the plant.

Most seeds do best if you soak them in water for a few hours before planting. You may want to soak my seeds and filled soil cups at the same time. Make certain that all of the products you will be using are well saturated with clean water.

The water that you use should be as free of chemicals as possible. If you have access to a clean stream or spring, this is an excellent place to obtain planting water. You could also collect rainwater to use in your garden. If necessary, most stores sell natural spring water.

After your seeds and soil are well moistened, you will sow the seeds. Most seeds do well with just a light covering of potting medium. A standard guide is to place the seed 3 times deeper than the size of the seed. Very tiny seeds are just barely placed into the soil while larger seeds are as much as ¼ inch into the medium.

Your seeds will need moisture protection during the early stages of development. You can purchase pre-made mini greenhouses or make a plastic tent to protect the seeds during germination and early development.

The seeds are now ready to do their job. You should place them in a warm area where they will not be disturbed. Seeds germinate at different paces so you will want to check on the seedlings often. A germinating seed requires warmth and moisture but does not need large amounts of light. Once the seedling emerges, it will require much more light.

If you are lucky enough to have a sunny area, natural light works well for most seedlings. Most indoor locations do not receive an adequate amount of light for new seedlings. You can use growing bulbs to provide light supplementation during the first weeks of seedling development. Each seedling will have varying light needs and you will want to check the exact growth requirements of the plants you have selected to grow.

A simple way to determine if your seedlings are getting enough light is to watch how they grow. Plants that are reaching for the light will begin to become leggy. That means they will grow tall, weak stems in an attempt to capture more light. If you notice your plants are growing tall but not thickening, chances are good that they are not receiving adequate light and you will need to add supplemental lighting.

Over the first few weeks, you will want to make sure that your seedlings stay moist but not saturated. The easiest way to keep the seedlings moist but not saturated is through bottom watering. If you have not already placed your growing cups on a tray, you will want to do so now.

The tray should have edges about as high as a cookie sheet. Pour water into the tray around the potting cups. This allows the soil to absorb the water that the plant needs through the drainage holes in a cup or through the cup itself if you are using biodegradable planting cups. Watering from the top increases the likelihood of washing the seeds too deeply into the soil or damaging the newly emerged plants.

Each morning and afternoon, check the water level in the seedling tray. If too much water remains in the bottom of the pan, you will need to lessen the amount you give at each watering. If the pan becomes dry too quickly, you will either need to give more water at each watering or water more frequently. The goal is to provide enough moisture to keep the soil damp but not soggy.

If you live in a very moist climate, you may want to remove the germinating plastic once the seedlings emerge. If you live in a dry climate, are propagating during a cold month, or are growing delicate plats, you may want to leave the germinating plastic on the plants until they have developed their second set of leaves. By the time the second set of leaves has developed, the root system is typically strong enough to support the plant. If you do choose to leave the moisture retaining cover on the plants, you will need to create vents to ensure that your seedlings and potting medium are not too wet.

Once the second set of leaves have developed on your seedling it is time to begin "hardening" the plant. If you are planning to transplant the seedling outdoors, hardening is a critical step. If you are planning to maintain an indoor garden, hardening is still important but not critical to the success of your seedling.

Hardening means giving your seedlings the opportunity to become strong enough to survive natural environmental changes. A nice first step to begin hardening your plants is to open a nearby window or allow a fan to blow close to but not directly at the plants. This gives the plants to chance to adapt to changes in airflow and temperature.

If the seedlings are going to be indoor plants, you can gradually increase the number of hours that they are exposed to the airflow.

If you will be transplanting the seedlings to an outdoor garden, you will need to adapt them to the outside conditions. Once they seem to be bearing up well to indirect air and alterations in temperature, you should take seedlings outdoors for a few hours at a time. Spend a week or two gradually increasing the amount of time the plants stay outdoors. Once they are spending most of the day outside and any chance of extremely cold temperatures or severe storms have passed, you can transplant the seedlings to their permanent home.

Select the strongest seedlings to transplant. Some people pull out the hardier seedlings for transplanting and give the less hardy seedlings a bit more time to strengthen while others simply discard the weaker seedlings. Both methods have their positive points so you should do what works best for your ultimate growing plans.

Before you plant your seedling, you will want to pinch off the lowest set or sets of leaves. These nodes will grow roots once the plant is placed in the soil.

You will pre-dig the holes for your seedlings whether you are planting them indoors or out. The hole should be deep enough to cover the bottom nodes you exposed when pinched the lower leaves. This deep planting will create a stronger plant and compensate for any legginess that the plants developed reaching for light as seedlings.

You will want to ensure that the transplant soil is free of chemicals, weeds, and other contaminants. You will also want to use the best potting soil for your seedlings. A good mixture is 1 part vermiculate, 1 part perlite and 1 part potting mix.

If you have planted the seedlings in biodegradable grow cups, you will likely pull out all of the weaker plants and place the grow cup in your prepared location.

If you have planted the seedlings in a home made grow cup, you will need to turn the cup to release the seedling for transplant. You should use care to not to tug on the stems or leaves when removing the plant from the cup. Pulling on the plant during transplant will harm the delicate structures that the plant needs to survive. You might need to use a knife to help release the plant and lever it out of the cup.

You might notice that the roots of the seedling are tightly bound in the shape of the planting cup. If the roots are tightly bound, you may want to loosen them before placing the plant into its permanent location. You can take your finger and gently tug the roots loose, as you would untangle long hair. You can also take a clean pair of gardening scissors and make a straight cut on the four sides of the root ball by beginning at the bottom and working toward your seedling. This process helps to agitate the roots and encourages new growth. It also helps to spread the roots so that they grow outward from the plant, penetrating the soil in every direction. Penetration in all directions helps to give your plant the highest potential for gathering nutrients and water from the surrounding soil.

After you have worked the roots, place the selected seedling into the prepared hole and backfill with the potting mixture you have selected. You will want to pat the soil around the plant to remove any air pockets. You may want to mulch around outdoor plants to help them retain moisture and to discourage weed growth.

Water the soil around the plants at least once a day for the first couple of weeks. The amount of water necessary will vary depending on the location, climate, type of plant, and soil conditions. The plants should stay moist but not soggy during the first weeks outdoors. Watering the soil instead of the plant helps to prevent damage to the seedling. Think of it as a method similar to the bottom watering you completed on your newly emerged seedlings.

Harvesting & Drying Herbs

One of the biggest questions about homegrown plants is when to harvest. Many plants can be harvested at the beginning of the flowering season, though some are better in the middle or end of the season. Each entry in the compendium gives a general idea on harvest times.

In general, if you are harvesting for the leaves or buds, you should harvest the plant before it blooms. If you are harvesting for the flowers & petals, you should harvest the plant in the middle of the growing season. If you are seeking seeds or roots, harvest them after the blooms have died off the herb.

If you observe your plants, you should be able to begin to recognize the peak time for harvesting. Like a ripe tomato, all plant parts have a point where they are perfect for harvesting. This peak point is when the scent is heaviest and the beneficial compounds are at the highest concentration.

The time of day that you harvest can change the success of the supplement you are making. Some plants are at their richest early in the morning while others become richer as the warmth and moisture of the day give them the strength that they need.

You will want to observe the specific type of plant that you are harvesting to determine what time of day might be the peak time for that plant. The default time to harvest when you are not sure is mid-morning. This is the time after the dew has evaporated but before the plants begin to wilt from the heat of the day.

You will decide how to harvest based on the type of plant, method of drying you plan, and ultimate use of the plants.

If you are primarily interested in only the flowers & leaves of the plant, you can pluck these off the mother plant and allow the remainder to continue growing in the hopes of getting another, larger harvest later in the season. If the plant is an annual or you need the roots, you will harvest the whole plant. If the plant is a perennial, you should use care not to over harvest since this increases the risk of killing the plant.

Once you have harvested the plant parts that you will use, you should clean them. If you have purchased plants from another grower, you will want to make certain any chemicals used during the growing process are cleaned off your plant parts. Even if you grow the plants yourself, you will want to wash the plants to remove any bugs, eggs, soil, and other contaminants that might have gotten in with your plants.

You can pat the plants dry with a clean, soft cloth or simply shake the excess water off the plant and allow them to finish drip-drying while you prepare whatever next step you will take with your plants.

One of the most common methods of using plants as supplements is as a dried product that will be made into teas, infusions, decoctions, or other products. The purpose of drying your plant products is to remove the fluids, preserve the beneficial compounds and extend the useful life of the plant parts.

There is some confusion related to using fresh or dried plant parts when making products like extracts, oil infusions, and other supplements. All fresh plant products will contain some amount of water. The type of plant part that you are using will dictate how much of the part is fluid and how much is plant. The presence of water will dilute the potency when you make supplements like an extract or tincture. You can use fresh plant parts but most people find that they attain a higher efficiency and need less storage room when they dry the plant matter before processing it into various supplements.

There are many ways to dry plant parts. Each of them has benefits and drawbacks. The three basic methods that are most often used for drying plants are air-drying, speed drying, and hang drying.

Air Drying

Air-drying is exactly how it sounds. You will expose the parts of the plant to the air to allow the moisture to evaporate. A few plants do well when air and sun are combined during the process but most should be kept out of direct sunlight since it can evaporate or damage the beneficial compounds you are drying the plant to obtain.

Air-drying is the slowest method of drying plant products but it may also help to retain more of the beneficial compounds.

Before starting the air-drying process, you should decide where you are going to dry the plants. If the weather is just right, you may be able to dry the plants outside away from direct sunlight and the weather. More often, you will want to select an area inside the home where the plant will not be disturbed during drying.

The biggest consideration is that the area you select must be very dry. Plants will not dry properly in a space with high humidity.

The second consideration is that the area should not get extreme air movement from nature or from fans, door closures, people, or another source. As the plant parts dry, they will become light. A good breeze will scatter the plants and ruin the project.

You should also consider the container you will use to dry your plants. There are many different types of air-drying racks available for purchase. Many of these allow you to stack the plants for drying. These are very convenient and some are even pretty. Depending on the amount of air-drying you will do, purchasing drying racks can become costly. If you want to keep costs low or will only be drying plants occasionally, you can make your own drying bins. A simple rack can be made by layering a clean cotton towel or waxed paper inside a shallow cookie sheet or even a cardboard box. Whatever bins you choose must not be able to absorb the compounds from your plant product, must not contaminate the plant product, must allow you to dry the plant parts in one layer not a pile, and must be durable enough to withstand the turning or agitation of the plant parts.

Once you have selected the container for your drying processes, you will need to finish preparing the plant products.

The cleaned, dried herbs will need to be broken down into smaller pieces. You can pull the leaves, flowers, and stems apart with your hands or use a pair of clean shears to achieve the right size.

Place the plant pieces into the prepared container in one thin layer. This helps ensure that more plant parts are exposed to the air. The more parts exposed to the air, the faster the plant materials will dry. The faster the plant materials dry, the less likely they are to develop mold growth.

Different plants will dry at different rates. You will want to agitate or turn your plant parts at least one time each day. The more moisture you have in the air or in the plant, the more frequently you will want to turn the mixture. The goal with agitating the plant parts is to ensure that everything dries evenly and quickly.

It is important that the plants dry as quickly as possible. If you enter a very humid period during the drying process, you may need to place the drying containers in the oven to help prevent excess moisture build up and possible mold growth.

Oven Assist

You can speed dry the plant products in the oven. This is not one of my favorite methods because you run the risk of cooking the plant parts instead of simply drying them. There are times when oven drying may be the only logical solution like when a high humidity day hits in the middle of the drying process. It may be a better choice to risk cooking the herbs rather than risk losing the entire batch to mold.

If you choose to use the oven assist drying method, you need to make certain that your oven is clean and free of chemicals. Any chemicals in the oven may pollute your plant products.

You should turn the oven on to its lowest setting and leave the door open to its first 'notch' or about 4 inches. This helps to allow air into the process and to keep the oven from becoming too warm.

You will need to array your plant parts as thinly as possible on the drying mat. A perforated oven-safe tray works best for oven assist drying. If you do not have an oven-safe tray, you can layer clean cotton or paper towels across the oven racks. Place the plant products onto the chosen holder.

The herbs will dry very quickly in the oven so you should check them every couple of minutes to ensure they do not over dry or 'cook'. The amount of time you will need to dry the plants will depend on the type of plant product you are using, the amount of moisture remaining in the plants, the humidity in the air, and other factors.

When you check the plants you will want to agitate them like you would during air-drying. This will help the plant parts to dry more evenly. If you are using a soft cloth and can safely pick it up, just bouncing the plant parts on the cloth a few times may be a sufficient method of agitation. If you are using a solid rack, turn the herbs every few minutes.

Speed Drying

Food Dehydrators have completely changed the way that some people dry their herbs. A dehydrator follows the same basic concept as air-drying it just does the job much more quickly. The dehydrator forces warm, dry air around the plant parts. This helps to remove the moisture from the plants more quickly and actually makes a more pleasing final product for some plant parts like oily fruit rinds, wood bark, and nut.

The dehydrator must have a fan and allow you to set the heat setting at its lowest setting or else you will cook your plant parts. If the dehydrator you are using has a recommendation in the manual for drying herbs, you should start with those instructions and then adapt the settings to suit your particular needs. If there are no recommendations, start the process with the temperature on the lowest setting, usually around 90°, and gradually increase the temperature if you feel the plants are drying too slowly.

You will spread the plant parts onto the dehydrator trays in a single layer. You should make your layer loose so that there is plenty of room for airflow to reach all sides of the plants.

The dehydrator will complete the drying process much more quickly than air-drying. You should check the plants every 15 – 20 minutes. At each check, you may want to rotate the trays. The plant parts closest to the heat source will dry more quickly and rotating the trays helps to distribute the airflow & heat. You should remove the plant parts as they become dry enough for use.

Hang Drying

Hang Drying is an easy way to dry herbs that works well if you have plenty of space and a controlled room where you can hang the plants. Hang drying also helps to produce a stronger final product when you are harvesting only the flowers & leaves.

You will want to be certain that there are no contaminants in the room for the plants to absorb during drying and that the air is very low in humidity. I use hang drying in the winter months since we have forced air heat that removes most of the humidity in air. It also helps to brighten and freshen the house naturally.

When you harvest for hang drying, you will leave longer stems on the plant parts. The stems will be used for the hanging. Cut each plant as close to the same length as you can.

Gather the ends of the stems together. You can use a pasta measure to judge how much you have gathered clumping about 1 serving worth per hanging group. If you make the hanging group too large, it will take longer to dry and you risk ruining the batch if the air cannot reach the middle plants.

Tie the gathered stems into a bouquet about 2 inches from the ends of your stems using natural string or jute. You will want to tie the stems tightly enough that they do not fall out of the clump but not so tightly that you break the stem. Leave an extra length of string to hook the clump to your hanger.

The stems will shrink as they dry so you may want to check the bundle occasionally to ensure that the tie has not loosened so much that you are losing stems.

Hang the herbs upside down with the cut stems facing toward the ceiling. This helps the compounds in the plant to travel toward the leaves & flowers strengthening the final product.

Hang drying makes seed capture easy if you plan to propagate a new batch of plants. Place a bin, paper bag, or cardboard box underneath the hanging plant. The bin will capture any plant parts or seeds that fall off when the plant becomes dry enough to release them.

The amount of time necessary for hang drying will depend on the temperature of the area, humidity in the air, moisture in the plant, density of the plant, and other factors. You should check the plants regularly to see if they are ready for storage.

Storing the Dried Product

Each plant product will dry at a different rate and you should check often to see if any of the matter is ready for use and storage. You will become adept at judging the progress of the drying by sight. You should be able to see & feel a gradual reduction in the moisture of the plant parts. In the beginning, there are certain signs you can look for to decide whether the plants are ready for storage.

Select a leaf or flower and hold them between your thumb and forefinger. Gently rub your fingers back and forth. The leaves & flowers will break into tiny pieces without much effort. They should not powder. If the plant parts powder as soon as you touch them, they are too dry. Over-drying the plant parts diminishes the power of the active compounds.

Select a berry or flower bud and look at it closely. It should look and feel like a hardened raisin.

Select a stem or twig that appears to be dry. Try to snap it into smaller pieces. Fully dried stems & twigs will snap easily much like a piece of uncooked spaghetti.

Select a nut or seed and place it on a hard surface like a cutting board. Attempt to crush it with a kitchen mallet, the bottom of a ceramic cup, or the side of your shears. Nuts & seeds should break into a powder that does not clump easily. If the powder is still clumping, there are likely too many oils in the nut or seed and you should allow them to dry further before storage.

If you are still not certain that the parts are ready for storage, you can select a small amount of the plant and place it in a clean, dry glass jar. Seal the lid tightly and place the jar in a warm, sunny location. If moisture condenses inside the jar over the first few hours, the plant is not ready for storage. If no moisture appears, the plant part is dry enough for storage.

You should store your newly dried plant product in a way that will not allow moisture or contaminants to permeate. Some people use special stainless storage cans while others make "bags" from waxed paper. Porcelain, ceramic, and glass are other common choices. You should choose whatever storage method works best in your household. Just select a storage container that blocks moisture, light, and chemical contaminants and your plants will retain much of their usefulness, ready for use when you need them though most should be used within 1 year of the harvesting date.

Freezing

Sometimes, plant parts need to be harvested at a time that is not conducive to drying or the parts just do not dry properly. When this happens, another option is to freeze the plants.

Some people make freezing their primary method of storage for all of their harvests. If you do not have a dry room, live in a moist climate, or are unable to air dry the plant parts for another reason, freezing may be an alternative.   You should remember that freezing is not technically a drying method and a great deal of the moisture will remain in the plant parts making any supplement made from freeze-dried plants weaker.

You will harvest and clean the plant parts the same way that you do in any storage process.

After the excess water has been removed, strip the leaves, petals, and any other plant parts that you plan to save. Place the usable pieces in the freezer storage container you have selected. The faster you freeze the parts the better so a deep freezer or the quick freeze shelf in some side-by-side freezers is a good choice. The plant parts should be good for 3-4 months.

Herbal Tea & Infusion

Once you have dried your plant parts, you will want to decide how to use your plants. Teas and infusions are two of the most common methods of using dried supplements. Making a natural tea or infusion allows you to obtain the benefits of the plants compounds while enjoying a variety of flavor sensations.

Infusions are not just for ingesting. You can use an infusion in the bath, in creams or lotions, as a wash, for cleaning, or for almost any other activity that can benefit from the compounds contained in the plants.

An infusion is made using the soft plant parts. These are parts like the flower or leaf.

You will need to decide the source of the water you will use to make your tea or infusion. Filtered water, spring water, and rainwater are all good sources. The primary concern with water is to ensure it has as few contaminates as possible.

You will want to choose a teapot or kettle for heating water that is not going to degrade and release chemicals into the final product. Glass, stainless steel, and ceramic are all common choices.

Warm the water to boiling in the kettle and then remove the water from the heat.

You will want to get a tea ball to contain your plant parts or tea strainer to help you remove the plant parts from the finished drink.

Tea balls tend to keep the plant parts together and leave far fewer 'clumps' in the finished drink but they also tend to compress the plant parts and make releasing the beneficial compounds more difficult.

Tea strainers allow the plant parts to move freely, releasing more of their compounds but also tend to allow small plant parts to escape into the finished drink.

Either option works well and the one that you choose will be based on your personal preference and needs.

You will choose the plant or combination of plant parts that provide the benefits you want from a supplement. These will vary greatly between people. You can even add a base tea just for the flavor! Regardless of the type of plants you are using, you will need between ¾ and 1 teaspoon of dried plant product per cup of liquid.

If you have not crumbled the plant parts before, you will want to break them into smaller pieces now. This gives the water more access to the plant parts and helps the compounds to release more easily.

You can add the dried pieces directly to your kettle as long as it has been removed from the heat source or place them in a cup and pour the water from the kettle on top.

Placing the herbs into the kettle, whether loose or in the tea ball, helps to prevent the oils from evaporating during steeping but also leaves residue behind that may interfere with the next supplement you make if you do not clean the kettle well after each use.

Pouring the water over the leaves in the cup allows more of the beneficial compounds to escape but helps to prevent cross contamination between supplement usages.

Either method of getting plant parts into contact with the water works and you should choose the option that suits you the best.

Allow the leaves to steep in the water for between 5 minutes and 6 hours depending on the supplement you are trying to create. A traditional tea is not as strong as an infusion and often an ingested supplement will be weaker than a topical preparation.

Once your drink is steeped to your desired strength, remove the plant parts from the liquid, flavor to taste and enjoy.

Cold Infusion

Many plants release their compounds best to warm water. Occasionally you may want to use a plant that does not release as well to heat. Some plants that are high in mucilage content or bitter compounds seem to do better when the compounds are infused in cold fluid. These are often referenced as digestive in descriptions.

A cold infusion is made by soaking the selected plant parts in room temperature or cooler liquid instead of hot water. You do not need to limit yourself to water. Some cold infusions are made with milk, juices, or another preferred liquid.

You will use the same proportions of plant parts and liquid as you do for a hot infusion. You will prepare the plant parts following the same processes. You will even consume the cold infusion the same way that you do a hot

171

infusion. The two major differences when making a cold infusion are that you will use cold water, milk, or another liquid instead of hot and you will allow the plant parts to steep for a longer period than you do with a warm infusion.

Decoction

A decoction is made with plant parts that are simmered in water. A decoction is usually used to extract the compounds from tougher plant parts like barks, roots, seeds, and wood. These plant parts are tougher than leaves or flowers and tend to require more heat to release the beneficial compounds.

The amount of plant product to water will vary depending on the plant you are using and the desired results. An average is 3 teaspoons of dried plant pieces for each 1 cup of water. You will want to adjust this ratio to suit the plant parts you are using and the results you need.

Tougher plant parts should be chopped finer when you begin. It is common to grate or powder decoction components before adding them to the water.

When making a decoction, you will simmer the plant parts instead of adding the plants to the water once it is already hot. This helps to force the tougher plants to release their compounds.

Add the plant parts and water to your simmering pot. A glass, stainless steel, or ceramic pot works well. You should place a lid on the pot to help prevent more loss of active compounds than necessary.

Simmer the decoction, keeping the heat just below a boil. The amount of time you will simmer the plant parts depends on a variety of factors including the plant's toughness and the strength you want from the finished product. Your goal is to reduce the fluids in the mixture. A traditional decoction is complete when the water has been reduced by ½. In other words, if you start with 1 cup of water, you will finish with ½ cup.

Strain the plant parts from the fluid as soon as you remove the mixture from the heat. Some decoctions may separate when cooled. Straining the plant parts while the mixture is hot allows you to retain the compounds. You may want to wear gloves and squeeze the excess fluids from the plant parts to reduce loss.

Since decoctions tend to be stronger than infusions because of the evaporation of some of the liquids, you will use less at a time. You can store extra liquids from your decoction in the refrigerator, often for 2-3 days depending on the plants that you have selected. You will want to store the decoction in a safe container like a stainless steel or glass bottle. Allow the mixture to cool before storage.

Shake or stir the decoction before each use. This ensures that any compounds that have separated are re-distributed.

Syrup

A decoction or infusion can sometimes be bitter or more liquid in nature than the treatment requires so it is a common practice to make it into a syrup product. This is especially true when dosing will be by the teaspoon or tablespoon instead of by the cup. Making an infusion or decoction into syrup may also help to extend the shelf life.

The amount of sweetener product like agave, sugar, or honey used to make syrup will vary depending on the personal preference of the user.

Traditional syrup is made using about 8 ounces of herbal fluid to 4 ounces of liquid honey, sweetener, or sugar. This amount will vary depending on personal preference and type of sweetener being used.

Heat the sweetener you have selected until it becomes liquefied. Remove the sweetener from the heat and add the plant infusion, powder, or decoction. Blend the ingredients well.

You may want to alter the mixture depending on the eventual use of the syrup. The thicker the syrup the better it "sticks". An example of a time when you want syrup to adhere well is if the syrup will be used as a treatment for a sore throat.

When you have attained the consistency you want, pour the finished syrup in a sterile, dark container. Refrigerating the syrup will help to extend the shelf life further. You can also add a natural preservative if you wish. Typical syrup will keep usable for between 8 to 16 weeks.

Electuary

The terms electuaries and syrups are used interchangeably by some people but are actually two different products. An electuary is a paste made of powdered plant products mixed with a base.

Powdered plant products are traditionally mixed with sweeteners like syrup, honey, berry jam or sugar and water. The powders and base are blended to make a paste product.

The plant products used to make an electuary should be powdered as finely as possible. A coffee grinder, food processor, or mortar and pestle all work well for powdering dried plant parts.

The composition of an electuary can be as basic as one part powdered plant product mixed with two parts honey and as complex as dozens of types of plant product mixed with multiple sweetening agents and carriers. Honey is a good choice as a base for many people since it can actually help to extend the usable life of the finished product. The powdered plants that are used will depend entirely on the supplement that you need. You can use as few or many plant powders and you want when making an electuary.

You will want to vary the balances of powder to carrier agent to suit your needs. Some powders are heavier and will require more carriers while others are lighter, and will need less. Common electuaries can range from 1 part powder to 3 parts carrier to 1 part powder to ½-part carrier.

When you have all of your components measured, heat the carrier or base slightly and blend in the powdered herbs. Store an unused electuary in a sterile, glass or metal container with a tight fitting lid.

Extract

An extract is a product made separating the active compounds of a plant product into a condensed state.   Extraction is traditionally accomplished using a solvent, expressing the compounds, or reducing a decoction to a thickened state.

Alcohol Extract or Tincture

An extract or tincture is made using plant parts and a solvent. Common solvents are grain alcohol, vodka, or wine. A simple explanation of the differences between extracts and tinctures is that an extract is traditionally made using 1 part plant matter to 1 part liquid while a tincture is made using 1 part plant matter to 3, 4, or even 5 parts liquid.

Alcohol extracts require three basic ingredients. You will need a glass or ceramic jar with a tightly fitting lid, a solvent like alcohol, and the desired plant products.

You will harvest and clean the plant parts according to the standard harvesting practices. Cut the plant parts into finely chopped pieces. You can use a blender or food processor to chop the plant parts. Make certain that you do not grind them into such fine pieces that you cannot strain the plant parts from the liquid when your extract is complete.

Place the plant parts into the jar. Fill the jar with the selected alcohol, making certain that all of the plant parts are covered.

There are commercially and traditionally established ratios of alcohol, water, and plant materials for each type of plant that you might process. You can refer to specific entries for the particular plant product or to commercial preparation standards to determine what is best for the particular plant you are extracting. In general, the higher the oil contents of the plant material, the higher the alcohol necessary to extract the oils.

Once the jar is filled, seal the jar. Shake the jar to agitate the materials and to ensure that as much of the plant product is in contact with the alcohol as possible. Place the jar in a cool, dark place where it will not be disturbed. Every morning and night, shake the jar to agitate the mixture and distribute the plant parts in the alcohol.

The amount of time that you will need to make an extract depends on the type of plant materials you are using. Soft leaves and petals yield more quickly than hard seeds & barks. Most extracts take between 2 and 8 weeks.

The final content of the alcohol extract should be approximately 25% alcohol. This helps to inhibit bacterial and fungal growth. Bacteria and fungus will still grow in an alcohol tincture but this ratio helps to slow the process.

When the extract has reached the strength you want, strain the plant products out of the liquid. You will want to squeeze all of the fluid out of the plant materials.

Alcohol extracts and tinctures should be stored away from light.

You can use a preservative to extend the shelf life of your tincture though it is not necessary. Some plant parts are natural preservatives.

Finished alcohol extracts or tinctures should be stored in dark glass containers to prevent the loss of active compounds over time. A finished alcohol extract will keep for as much as 3 years.

Expressed Extract

You can make an expressed extract by pressing the juice out of certain types of plant parts. Not all plants can be juiced. If you are working with a plant part that can be juiced, you will express the liquid from the part using a plant press, juicer, or simply by squeezing the applicable part.

Some juices can be used as a remedy in their own right. You will want to save every usable part of the plants you buy, grow, or harvest.

Typical extract treatments would use the plant part that is left after the excess juices are expressed. You will apply the plant parts to the affected area or prepare it according to the supplement instructions for ingestion.

Simmer Extract

Some extracts are made through simmering. Much like a decoction, you will simmer the plant parts to condense it down to its most potent form. Extracts can be made using oil, alcohol, vinegar, or water. You will follow the same steps as you do when making a decoction but you will reduce the fluid to ¼ or less of its original liquid volume. In other words, if you start with 1 cup of fluid, you will finish when you have ¼ cup of fluid.

Infusion Flavoring

Sometimes the flavor of liquids like vinegar, oils, and alcohol can be enhanced by the addition of plant parts. Infusion flavorings provide not only the flavor and aroma but also the compounds of the plant parts selected for the process.

Alcohol Infusion

Flavored alcohol has become very popular in recent years. You can make your own flavored, custom blends at home and add beneficial compounds customized to your specific wants & needs.

You can make flavored alcohol infusions using the same barks, flowers, fruits & leaves that you use to make your other products. Many available recipes include popular flavor combinations. You can use these if you just want to make flavored cocktails. Since this is all about obtaining the benefits of plant products, you may want to experiment with your own custom blends that not only taste great but also provide the healthy supplemental benefits that suit your personal situation.

You can make an alcohol infusion out of almost any liquor but most people prefer vodka. Vodka has a neutral flavor that can easily be changed through plant infusions. Rum, gin, whiskey, almost any alcohol that you prefer will take flavor from a plant infusion. Select the alcohol that suits your preferences.

The biggest difference in this type of infusion is that fresh flowers, fruits, leaves, and other parts work better than the dried variety when making a flavored infusion. You will clean the plant parts you have selected. You should remove any damaged or spoiled pieces. You will also want to remove and discard any plant parts you do not want in your final product. For example, if you are using berries as part of your mixture, you may want to remove any leaves and stems attached to the berry. These will have different properties and give the final infusion a different taste.

You will need to chop or grind the plant parts. The finer you chop the plant parts, the better the flavor will infuse. Unless you are using the plant parts as a dressing, you will not want to chop them so fine that they are difficult to remove from the finished product.

The amount of plant parts to alcohol you are using, the exact plant parts you select, and the flavor you want from your finished product. A good guideline is ½ part plant parts to 1 part alcohol. You can adjust this as you become more familiar with the flavors of the plant parts you select.

Since this recipe is not dealing with very specific ingredients but rather generalities of processes, it is impossible to predict exactly what the balance will be for your particular recipe. Some plant products like juicy fruits yield flavor more quickly than some tougher plant products like nuts. You may need more alcohol to extract the flavor or less depending on exactly what you are using and exactly how you want your drink to taste.

Seal the infusion jar with a tight fitting lid and place it in a warm area of your home. Some people find that the flavor infuses more quickly when the jar is placed in a sunny location. This may lower the beneficial effects of the plant compound but since flavored alcohol is as much about taste as it is about benefits, you may want to consider using sunlight as a tool. A more pure method of infusing is to keep light away from the mixture to help protect as many of the beneficial compounds as possible.

No matter what plant products you are using as a flavoring, you will want to keep a close taste watch on your infusion. The flavor is going to be custom suited to your tastes so sample a few drops of the infusion every couple of days. When the flavor mix reaches your preference, the infusion is done. If the flavor mix becomes too strong, you can always dilute it with extra alcohol.

After your flavor has reached its peak, you will strain the plant parts from the alcohol base. A coffee filter, cheesecloth, or fine kitchen strainer all work well for removing plant parts.

Store the liquid in a clean, airtight container and enjoy. Just remember that you have transferred the active compounds of the plant parts into your alcohol and read the maximum daily limits and potential side effects before using your new product.

Vinegar Infusion

Many people enjoy the flavor and aroma of a custom vinegar blend. Flavored vinegars are made following the same processes as flavored alcohol. You simply replace the alcohol with vinegar.

There are two important considerations regarding infused vinegar that you should remember. The vinegar will contain the compounds of the plants used during the process. Most people tend to use vinegar more freely in the family diet than they do alcohol. You should always review the potential effects, good and bad, of any plant materials before adding them to your diet. The infused vinegar will also be prone to the same type of spoilage as any other vinegar product.

OILS

Oil Extracts, Oil Flavorings, and Essential Oils are very different products. Each of them can be made at home but they do require slightly different processes. The processes for aromatic, supplement, and flavored oils are similar to making other supplements & flavorings. The differences between one method of extraction and the next is the strength of the finished product.

Cold Oil Infusion

An oil infusion is used to extract the oil soluble compounds in plant parts for use as a flavoring, aroma element, and supplement product.

You can infuse oil using the same processes you would use for alcohol and vinegar flavorings. You will harvest, clean, and prepare the plant parts that you want in your oil according to the standard harvest instructions. Many people find that dried plant parts work better in oil infusions than fresh plant parts. Dried plant parts have had most of the water removed from the plant and may blend better than fresh.

You should select the oils that work best for your personal situation and your taste preference. Olive oil is the most commonly selected flavored oil base but other oils work equally well. If you will be using your oil as a supplement instead of a flavoring, you will want to modify the oil selection accordingly.

When making the oil infusion, follow the alcohol infusion instructions but replace the alcohol with oil. Just like with any infusion, it is important to remember that the flavored oil will contain the active compounds of the plant parts you selected. Make certain that you use oil according to the correct daily dosing limits and consider the potential effects of the plant parts before serving the oil product to others.

Sun Oil Bath

One of the most common methods of extracting essential oils from a plant is to use an oil bath. You will select the plant materials to be used. Chop them into fine pieces. Place the chopped materials in a glass jar. Add a carrier oil with a long shelf life like jojoba until the plant matter is completely covered. Seal the jar and place it in the sun.

Direct sunlight may heat the oils too much so you should select an area that receives diffused sunlight. Windowsills are the most commonly chosen location. Allow the oil bath to heat throughout the day. Shake the jar each night to speed the process.

Continue to allow the oil bath to extract the essence until you feel that no further progress is being made. Strain the plant materials out of the oils. The resulting oil will not be as strong as the oils you obtain through distillation or solvent extraction.

You can re-infuse the oils to make them stronger. Simply repeat the process using the same oils as you did during the first sunbath but use fresh plant products. Each time you repeat the process with the same oil, the result will be stronger.

The stronger the oil becomes, the higher the likelihood of a reaction. You should make sure that you protect your skin from the oils and plant parts to minimize the likelihood of irritation.

Using Infused Oils

Infused oils are frequently used in culinary and supplemental preparations. Infused oils are also used to make lotions, creams, and other topical preparations. You can find a variety of natural product recipes for the hair, lips, nails and skin. The infused oils that you have made using the appropriate plant parts can be used in replacement for the liquid in your selected recipe.

There are two important considerations regarding infused oils that you should remember. The oils will contain the compounds of the plants used during the process. You should always review the potential effects, good and bad, of any plant materials before adding them to your diet. The infused oils will also be prone to the same type of spoilage as any other oil product.

Essential Oils

An essential oil is much stronger than infused oil. When you make an oil infusion, you are diluting the compounds with the alcohol, vinegar, or oil base. When making an essential oil, you are capturing the concentrated plant essences in their pure form and not diluting the results.

Essential oils are most frequently used for topical and aromatherapy treatments. Essential oils are often very powerful and should not be applied directly to the skin. Essential oils must be diluted before use.

The method of extraction that you use to garner essential oils will depend on the specific plant, ultimate use, and desired strength of the oil.

Distillation

The most common method of commercial essential oil extraction is by distillation. Distillation uses water to help extract the oils. There are different methods of distillation. You can purchase a distillation unit for personal use, make your own distillation unit using a pressure cooker and tubing, or you can use one of the more common home methods of extraction like solvents.

Steam Distillation

Steam distillation uses a source of steam piped into the distillation unit at a high pressure. The steam passes through the plant material and exits into a condenser unit. The product in the condenser unit is the plant essence or essential oil.

Steam distillation units can be purchased or you can make your own steam distillation unit from a pressure cooker, tubing, and capture jar. These unites are somewhat complex and you will want to review commercial distillation units and homemade distillation unit creation instructions before attempting to make a unit of your own.

Hydro-Distillation

Hydro-Distillation is extraction accomplished by covering the plant materials in water. You can envision it as being similar to making a soup. The water is heated to produce a steam that contains the plant essence. The steam is captured and used in therapeutics. This method works well for tougher materials like nuts, wood, and roots.

Hydro-Distillation units are similar to standard steam distillation units and can be purchased for in home use.

Tray Distillation

A tray distillation is much like the process that you would use to steam vegetables for food. The plant material is placed into a sieve like pan. The sieve is then placed over another pan filled with water. A tightly fitting lid with a tube leading out of it is placed on top. The water is boiled so that the steam passes through the plant material. The concentrated liquid is captured and piped through the tube to the holding unit. This method of distillation works best for soft plant materials. These units are also available for purchase.

Simmer Extraction

You can simmer extract compounds from plant products. This does use more heat and runs the danger of destroying the very compounds you want to protect, but it is a quick and simple method of extracting scented, essential oils at home.

You will select the base oil that you want to use for your simmer. The type of oil you select will depend largely on the ultimate use you will make of your essential oils. If you are using the oils in skin care, massage treatments, or other topical preparations then you will want to select oil that is compatible with your skin type. If you will use your oils in aromatherapy treatments, you will want to select neutral oil that diffuses well.

Prepare your plant materials by chopping, grinding, or pounding the plant parts. Once again, the more parts of the plant that you expose to the oils, the better the extraction results.

Put the prepared plant parts in the pot you will use for heating. Some people like to use a crock-pot while others prefer to use a saucepan. Either will yield approximately the same results so the choice is a matter of personal preference.

Add enough of the selected carrier oil to cover the plant materials.

Cover the pan with a tight fitting lid.

Most people find that they have better results and improve the likelihood of success if they use a water bath to heat the oils. Select a pan that is larger and deeper than the pan you have chosen for your plant & oil mixture. Fill this pan with 2-3 inches of water. Place the plant & oil pan into the water bath pan.

Heat the oil and plant mixture to a temperature between 100° and 125°. Do not overheat the oil bath because you will cook the plants instead of extracting the compounds.

Allow the mixture to simmer, stirring occasionally for 3 to 4 hours. You should make certain that you do not reduce the oil amount when you stir the plants. Evaporation may cause some of the oils to escape. You want to minimize evaporation.

Remove the mixture from the heat source. You can strain the plant materials from the oil immediately or allow the plant & oil mixture to continue to steep. Some plants & oils can steep for weeks and retain some active compounds while others will yield all of the available compounds during the heating process. You will need to get to know the plant materials that you have selected. It is important to experiment to learn how the plant parts will react to different processes. Generally, the softer the plant materials, the more quickly they yield the compounds.

It is recommended that you use rubber gloves to protect your skin when working with essential oils. The stronger the essential oils, the more likely they are to cause a reaction.

Strain the oils through cheesecloth. Squeeze any remaining oil out of the plant materials. Discard the leftover plant materials.

You can repeat the process with new plant materials and the oil that you gathered from the first extraction. Each repeated extraction with the same oil will increase the potency.

Solvent Extraction

Some plant essences cannot survive the heat distillation methods. These will require cold extraction. You can use a solvent to extract the essential oils through cold methods.

Select the plant materials that contain the highest amount of active scent compounds. Chop, grind, or bruise the plant materials as appropriate for the types of plant parts you have selected. Place the chopped and bruised plant material on a tray with perforations. A dehydrator tray works well. Place the tray over a capture pan.

You will use a solvent like grain alcohol or hexane to extract the matter from the plant. The solvent will extract everything that is dissolvable in the plant including waxes, pigments, and the aromatic oils.

You can use the solvent as a wash. To do this, you must have a capture pan that sits below the perforated plant tray. Pour the solvent over the plant materials. Remove the resulting liquid from the capture tray and pour it over the plant products again. Continue this process until the wash produces little or no new extraction.

You can also use the solvent as a bath. To do this, you must have a capture pan that allows the perforated tray to sit inside of it. Place the plant materials on the perforated tray. Sit the tray inside the capture pan. Pour the solvent over the plants until they are just covered. Allow the bath to sit, stirring occasionally. The length of time you must allow the bath to sit will depend on the plant material. Each plant material will give up the essences at a different pace. You can agitate the plant product occasionally to speed the process. When you believe that there is no longer any matter left to be extracted, remove the plant materials from the bath. Strain any remaining solid matter from the liquid.

When you have removed the solid matter, place the liquid into a container and seal it. The liquid should not completely fill the container. You should keep at least ¼ of the space in the container empty to allow for expansion later.

Allow the mixture to rest for a day or two. You will note that the materials separate. You should be able to view three layers.

You will have an opaque or thick layer of impurities. This layer will either fall to the bottom of the jar or lay on the top of the mixture.

The solvent alcohol will appear neutral.

You will see a layer that contains the oil essences. This layer will not appear as polluted as the impurity layer or as clear as the alcohol layer. This is your essential oil layer.

When your layers have formed, carefully lift the jar without agitating the layers. Loosen the lid to prevent breakage as the materials expand. Place the jar in the freezer. The oils and impurities will freeze. The alcohol will not freeze.

Place the entire frozen mass on a straining board. If the materials have frozen to the jar, you can gently separate them with a stainless steel knife.

The alcohol will drain away. Capture the alcohol in another jar as it strains away. You will want to freeze the alcohol again to gather any remaining oils that did not separate during the first freeze.

If the oils and impure layer are next to each other, use a knife to separate the usable oils from the impurities. Discard the impurities.

Place the frozen mass of oils onto a cheesecloth spread over a capture bowl or jar. As the mixture thaws, the oils will strain into the bowl. Anything that remains in the cheesecloth is plant material that was missed during the first straining. This can be discarded. The oils that strain into the bowl are the essential oils. Place the finished essential oils into your final storage jars.

The alcohol that you set aside earlier should be returned to the freezer for a second time. Any oils that remain in the solvent will freeze.

When the oils have frozen, remove the jar from the freezer and strain it through cheesecloth spread over an empty capture bowl. The alcohol will drain through the cheesecloth leaving the frozen oil behind. You can discard the alcohol or save it for use in your next extraction. Do not use the alcohol to extract the oils from a different type of plant material unless you have considered the active compounds of both types of plant materials.

The frozen oil parts should be allowed to thaw into another jar. The cheesecloth will filter any residual plant solids that remain. Add the captured oils to the essential oil jar you created during the first separation.

Store the essential oils in a cool, dark area for maximum shelf life.

Cold Pressing

Cold pressing works well for citrus peels and other plant parts whose oils can be released by scoring the plant product. You will score the plant, press the body and capture the oils being released.

External Use of Plant Products

Plant products can also be used as traditional topical preparations. There are numerous ways of using plant products in external preparations. You can use plant products in cleaners, washes, ointments, salves, creams, poultices, lotions and so forth. Any topical preparation you purchase at the store can be made from scratch using plant products.

There are numerous natural product recipe guides available, including my Green & Natural book series that include simple recipes that you can create to replace almost every product that you use. You can also create your own custom topical preparations using the plants detailed in the compendium.

The following explanations will help you to gain a fundamental picture of some of the most common topical preparations and the steps necessary to create them yourself.

Fomentation & Compress

A fomentation is the use of a strong herbal infusion externally as a compress.

If you are using soft plant parts, you will follow the infusion instructions but allow the plant parts to steep for a longer period than you would when creating a drinkable infusion.

If you are using hard plant parts, you will follow the instructions from making a decoction but reduce the fluid to 1/3 or even ¼ of the original fluid amount.

Once the infusion or decoction has reached the desired strength, you will soak a clean cloth in the liquid. Cotton and wool are common fabric choices for fomentations. The saturated cloth is then applied to the affected part.

You should use most fomentations while still hot. In general, you want the fomentation to be as hot as can be handled. When the cloth cools, saturate it in the fluid again and reapply to the affected area. You may want to use two cloths. One is applied while the other is soaking in the hot liquid.

Most fomentations can be wrapped in clean plastic and an elastic bandage to help retain the heat and to keep moisture from getting all over everything nearby.

You will continue to apply the fomentation according to the instructions of the plant parts that you are using and condition that you are treating. The time usage of a fomentation could range from less than an hour to a couple of days treatment. Gently re-heat the fomentation when it becomes too cool to use.

Some conditions do not lend themselves to hot heat. If the patient, conditions, or other reason makes hot heat undesirable, the fluid can be used as a cool compress. You will follow the same instructions as you would when making a fomentation, but you will allow the mixture to cool before applying it to the skin. When the compress becomes too warm, you will exchange it for a fresh, cool cloth.

Poultice

A poultice is made by chopping, bruising, or grating plant parts into smaller parts and applying them directly to an injured, inflamed, or problem area. The size of the plant parts used will vary depending on the instructions relating to the specific plant, malady, and supplement.

Some poultices are made by cutting the plant so that the internal parts are exposed and applying the product directly to the skin. An example of this type of poultice is the use of an aloe leaf to sooth a burn.

Other poultice recommendations require you to nearly powder the plant parts and mix the product with a small amount of water to form a paste.

The method of application will depend on the plant product and condition you are trying to alleviate.

Some poultices are hot preparations. A hot poultice is most often used to increase blood flow, alleviate pain, reduce inflammation, and relax muscles.

Hot poultices can be made by adding hot water to the ground plant parts to form a paste and applying the paste to the affected area.

A few plant parts should be directly heated before applying them to the area to be treated. You should use caution when heating plant parts because overheating can destroy beneficial compounds.

The most common method of making a hot poultice is to layer the plant parts on the area to be treated. You will then cover the plant parts with a moist, hot cloth. This method helps to increase the heat and lengthen the time of the treatment. The cloth is moistened and heated, usually using the microwave or the steam from a pan of boiling water. The cloth is exchanged for a warm one as it cools.

Some poultices are cold preparations. Cold Poultices are traditionally used to draw heat or toxins from an area, reduce congestion, and as a counter to hot poultices in cases of painful inflammation. Common uses of a cold poultice are in treating skin sores, ulcers, wounds, and skin conditions like eczema.

When creating a cold poultice, you will wet the plant parts with room temperature to icy cold fluid as indicated by the plant parts being used and condition being treated. The cold compress is then traditionally applied directly to the area being treated.

Poultices occasionally call for a plant part that is irritating to the skin. If the necessary plant parts include skin irritants, you should use a thin layer of cloth between the skin and the poultice. This will not allow for concentrated absorption of beneficial compounds but it will protect the skin from damage while still providing some benefit.

It is important to remember that using plant parts as a topical preparation still delivers the compounds of the plant into the body. The skin is the largest organ in the body and it readily absorbs compounds that are placed into direct contact with it. You can overuse a poultice.

Ointment

An ointment is made by blending powdered plant parts, plant decoctions, plant extracts, or plant oils into a base. Ointments generally contain oils, thickeners, hardeners, and plant parts. Ointments do not usually contain water.

When making ointments you will need a base, the preferred plant parts, and sterile containers. You may also choose to use a thickening agent, hardener, and preservative depending on the type of application, storage length, and slip desired in the product.

The base or carrier can be a liquid substance like almond oil, jojoba, or Vitamin E oil or semi liquid like cocoa butter or lanolin. These carriers each have properties, benefits and side effects of their own. You will want to consider the potential effects of the carrier when making your selection.

The oily, liquid carriers are commonly used in massage lotions and for creating topical pain-relief rubs. These can be made into a thicker ointment by incorporating a thickening agent and a hardener into the recipe.

The semi-solid carriers like cocoa butter tend to be used in products meant for application in a thin layer like in skin condition preparations. These can still be blended with thickening agents and hardeners but it is often not necessary.

Depending on the use of your finished product, the recipe may benefit from a hardener. The need for a hardener depends on the application method you plan for your product. The most common hardeners are waxes like beeswax and paraffin wax.

Some ointments will be used very quickly and are designed to treat a short-term issue. Others may be used over a period of weeks or months. If you plan to use the ointment over a period of weeks, you will want to add a preservative. Some plants have natural preservative properties while others will require enhancement. You should review the compendium to decide what type of preservative will work best with your particular recipe.

Gather all of the materials you have decided will work well in your recipe.

Most ointments are oil based. You will want select the appropriate oil base for your particular need. You will also find that using powdered or oil extracted plant components makes blending the ointment easier. Water based extractions or infusions do not blend as easily and may require the additional of an emulsifier.

Use a water bath to heat any carrier oil, thickening agents and hardener you plan to incorporate into your recipe. You should not heat the plant parts because heat may destroy the beneficial components.

When the carrier oil, thickener and hardening agents are warmed to a liquid state, whip them into the plant materials you have prepared.

Immediately, pour the resulting mixture into a clean tub, jar, or tube.

Seal the container and add the appropriate label.

Depending on the exact ingredients you have used, shake well before each use of the lotion or ointment. Ointments that contain thickeners and hardeners will not need to be shaken as much as those that do not.

Labeling

If you are only making one type of plant product, you will probably remember what is in the jar or bag. Chances are good that you will not be able to stop with just one. Once you realize how easy and satisfying making your own natural products can be, you will probably make many different products intended for many different supplements and uses. This makes labeling an important part of the process.

There is certain information that I find invaluable

Date Started
Plants Included
Plant parts used
Amount
Base – oils, alcohol, vinegar, etc
Amount
Date Completed – Storage Date
Expiration Date

You will want to continue to explore the many, many uses of plant products. This recipe guide gives you a wide range of products that you can make and use today. My compendium provides an in-depth look at a larger variety of traditional plants used by herbalists in the past. Scientific and natural research is constantly being done to fine tune our knowledge of the potential of plants. There are many, many sources of plant knowledge, recipes, and product creation guides available. I hope that this guide has given you a healthy knowledge base and a basic understanding of the potential uses of the plants you see every day. Feel free to drop me a note telling me about your new discoveries, recipes that you love, or just to say hi! There is nothing more satisfying than sharing my love of plants and nature with a fellow creator.

Appendix – Glossary

Abortifacient – is a substance that is capable of inducing an abortion

Adaptogenic – is a substance that has a normalize effect against changes brought about by stressors

Alopecia – A condition where hair is lost or partially lost from a place where it normally grows also called baldness.

Amenorrhea – refers to the absence of normal menstruation.

Analgesic - is a pain-killing drug or medicine.

Anocyne - is a pain-killing drug or medicine.

Antibacterial – is a substance that is active against bacteria.

Anti-Convulsant – is a substance used to reduce or prevent convulsions.

Anti-Emetic – is a substance that reduces or prevents nausea or vomiting.

Anti-Fungal – is a substance that alleviates or prevents fungal infections.

Antihistamine - is a substance that inhibits the physiological effects of histamine. Histamine is the chemical released by the body during an allergic reaction.

Anti-Inflammatory – is a substance used to reduce inflammation.

Anti-Microbial- is a substance that kills or inhibits the growth of microorganisms

Anti-Oxidant – is a molecule that inhibits the oxidation of other molecules.

Anti-Periodic – is a substance used to treat malarial-type symptoms or to prevent the recurrence of malarial like symptoms.

Anti-Parasitic – is a substance used to treat or prevent parasitic infestations.

Anti-Septic – is a substance capable of preventing or treating infection by inhibiting the growth of microorganisms.

Anti-Spasmodic - is a substance that suppresses muscle spasms.

Antitussive – is a substance used to suppress or relieve coughing.

Anti-Viral – is a substance that prevents or treats viral infections by killing a virus or that suppresses its ability to replicate.

Aphrodisiac – is a substance that stimulates sexual desire.

Aromatic – is a substance having a pleasant and distinctive smell that is used as a treatment.

Aroma Therapy – is the process of using an aromatic plant extract or essential oil to cause a physical or psychological effect in treatments.

Aspergillus – is a type of common mold that cause food spoilage and potentially disease.

Astringent - is a substance that causes the contraction of body tissues.

Botanical Name – is the Latin name give to a species of plant to distinguish it from other plants.

Bursitis – is a condition where there is inflammation in the bursa – elbow, knee, shoulder.

Cardiac – refers to the heart.

Carminative – is a substance that relieves flatulence.

Cathartic - is a purgative substance.

Cholagogue - is a substance that stimulates the secretion of bile from the gallbladder.

Coagulant - is a substance that causes blood to clot or coagulate

Colorant - is a substance that colors something usually food, cosmetics, or textile products.

Common Name – is the non-specific name used for everyday reference to a plant

Comminution – is the action of reducing a material or substance. When processing plants the act of reducing the size of the plant parts by cutting, grinding, or pounding

Conjunctivitis – is an infection or irritation causing inflammation, itching, and redness of the white part of the eye.

COPD – stands for Chronic Obstructive Pulmonary Disease, which is a disorder that involves constriction of the airways and difficulty breathing.

Decoction – is the result of concentration the essence of a substance or plant part by heating or boiling.

Demulcent – is a substance that soothes inflammation and protects irritated internal tissues.

Depurative – is a substance that facilitates the removal of impurities or cleansing of bodily fluids.

Detoxification - is the process of removing toxic substances or qualities from matter.

Diaphoretic – is a substance that induces perspiration.

Diosgenin – is a steroid compound used in the synthesis of steroid hormones.

Diuretic – is a substance causing increased passing of urine.

Dram – is a unit of measurement equaling approximately 1/16 of a dry weight ounce in US measurement 1/8 of a fluid ounce in Apothecary measurement.

Dysmenorrheal – refers to menstruation with excessive pain involving abdominal and lower back cramping.

Emetic - is a substance that causes vomiting.

Emmenagogue – is a substance that stimulates or increases menstrual flow.

Emollient – is a substance that has a softening or soothing affect on the skin.

Estrogenic – is a substance acting like, relating to, or caused by estrogen.

Expectorant – is a substance that promotes the secretion of mucus from the air passages.

Expression – is the process of forcibly separating liquids from solids.

Febrifuge – is a substance used to reduce fever.

Fluid extract – is a type of fluid-solid substance obtained from plant matter through water or alcohol processing

Galactagogue - is a substance that stimulates milk secretion.

Glycosides – is a compound formed from a simple sugar and another compound by the replacement of a hydroxyl in the sugar molecules.

Gram-Positive Bacteria – is a class of bacterial that are stained dark blue or violet by gram staining including bacteria such as pneumococci, staphylococci, and streptococci.

Gram Negative Bacteria - A class of bacterial that do not retain the stain used in gram staining including bacteria such as e. coli, shingella, and salmonella.

Hallucinogenic – is a psychoactive substance capable of producing hallucinations or altered sensory experiences.

Hepatic – refers to being of or relating to the liver.

Hydration – is the process of combining with or giving water.

Hypoallergenic – is a substance unlikely to cause an allergic reaction.

Hypoglycemic – is a condition indicated by low blood sugar.

Hypotensive – is a condition of abnormally low blood pressure.

Histamine – is the chemical released by the body during an allergic reaction.

Immuno-Stimulant - is a substance that stimulates the immune system to fight infection.

Infusion – Aqueous – is a drink or extract made by soaking plant parts in water.

Infusion – Oil – is a drink, extract, or product made by soaking plant parts in oil.

Insecticide - Substance used for killing insects.

Interferon - is a protein released in response to a virus that has the ability to inhibit virus reproduction.

Laxative – is a substance that stimulates or facilitates evacuation of the bowels

Lipase – is an enzyme that facilitates the breakdown of fats to fatty acids and glycol to other alcohols.

Maceration – is the process of softening plant materials by soaking or steeping in a liquid. To separate the compounds by soaking or steeping

Menorrhagia – refers to abnormally heavy menstrual bleeding.

Menstruum - is a solvent or mix of solvents.

Microphage – is a cell found in the tissues or at the site of an infection that takes in foreign material.

Mordant – is a substance that combines with a dye or stain to fix the colorant into a material.

Muscle Relaxant – is a substance that reduces muscle tone or contractibility.

Narcotic – is a psychoactive substance affecting mood or behavior.

Nervine – is a psychoactive substance that calms the nerves.

Nutritive – is a substance that is nutritious or provides nourishment.

Percolation – is the extraction of soluble components by passing the liquid through a filtering medium.

Pharynx – is the membrane-lined cavity behind the nose and mouth that connects them to the esophagus.

Phytoestrogen – are compounds found in plants that can mimic the effects of estrogen.

Pleurae – is the membranes lining the thorax and enveloping the lungs.

Pleurisy – is an inflammation of the pleurae that causes pain when breathing.

Polysaccharide – is a carbohydrate that is a compound of sugar molecules bonded together.

Proof Spirit – is a mixture of alcohol and water containing 50% alcohol by volume standard in the US.

Purgative – is a substance that is strongly laxative in effect.

Pulmonary – relates to the pulmonary system.

Phytosterol – is a group of naturally occurring steroid plant compounds.

Reparative – is a substance that helps to repair.

Rhinitis – is the inflammation of the mucus membrane of the nose.

Rubefacient – is a substance whose external application produces increased circulation or redness of the skin.

Saponins – is a class of steroid and terpenoid glycosides that are used in detergents and foams when shaken with water.

Sciatica – refers to nerve pain caused by compression of a spinal nerve in the lower back that affects the back, hip, or leg.

Sedative – is a substance that causes a calming or sleep-inducing effect.

Squalene – is an oily liquid that is the precursor to sterols.

Sterols – is a naturally occurring unsaturated steroid alcohol.

Steroidal – relates to steroid hormones or their effects.

Stimulant – is a substance that raises levels of physiological or nervous activity in the body.

Styptic – is a substance that causes bleeding to stop.

Succus – refers to several liquids in the body commonly termed digestive juices but also to the juice of fresh plant material.

Tincture – is a substance made by dissolving plant materials in alcohol.

Vasodilator – is a substance that causes dilation of blood vessels.

Vermifuge – is a substance that destroys parasites.

Viscosity – is the resistance of a liquid to movement and flow.

www.ingramcontent.com/pod-product-compliance
Lightning Source LLC
Chambersburg PA
CBHW082354270326
41935CB00013B/1624